About the Author

The author grew up in the West Midlands, the youngest of seven children to loving parents, John and Sandra. In a household bustling with the constant energy of siblings, finding quiet moments to nurture his passion was both a challenge and a necessity. His passion was always to write, a calling that seemed to emerge from the very fabric of our chaotic yet warm family life.

THE WEIGHT OF STONES

Carl.M.Holton

THE WEIGHT OF STONES

Vanguard Press

VANGUARD PAPERBACK

A CIP catalogue record for this title is available from the British Library.

ISBN 978-1-83671-973-1

Vanguard Press is an imprint of
Pegasus Elliot Mackenzie Publishers Ltd.
www.pegasuspublishers.com

First Published in 2026

Vanguard Press
Sheraton House Castle Park
Cambridge England

Printed & Bound in Great Britain

Chapter One
Mary

The morning Mary Costello was born, her mother died screaming curses at the midwife, at God, and at the husband who had put another child in her belly when she was already worn thin as parchment from bearing five others. The cottage reeked of blood and death, and when the infant finally drew breath, it was air thick with her mother's final words, words that would echo in the thatched walls long after the body was carried out and buried in the hard Irish earth.

Mary's father, Seamus Costello, looked upon his newborn daughter with the same expression he might have given a runt pig or a cow gone dry. She was the sixth mouth to feed in a household that could barely sustain three, and worse still, she was a girl, useless for the heavy work of farming, destined only to drain his meagre resources until some other man might take her off his hands. If any man would have her at all, given the circumstances of her birth and the poverty that clung to the Costello name like bog mist.

The other children, four boys and one girl, regarded their new sister with a mixture of resentment and indifference. There was no celebration, no blessing from the priest, no gathering of neighbours to welcome another soul into the world. Mary simply existed, a burden that had cost them their mother and would continue to cost them in ways both seen and unseen.

From her earliest memories, Mary understood that she was unwanted. While her brothers received what little affection their father could spare, she was left to fend for herself among the chickens and pigs in the yard. Her sister, Brigid, five years her senior, had inherited their mother's bitter tongue and their father's cruel disposition. She delighted in reminding Mary daily that she was the reason their mother lay cold in the churchyard, that she was a curse upon the family, that she would have been better left to die with the woman who bore her.

The cottage where Mary spent her childhood was little more than a hovel, its walls built of stacked stones and mud, its roof a patchwork of thatch that leaked in a dozen places when the rains came. There was one room for all seven of them, with a dirt floor that turned to mud in winter and baked hard as stone in summer. The fire in the centre provided their only warmth and light, and around it they huddled like animals, fighting for space and scraps.

Seamus Costello was a man broken by poverty and loss, but he had not always been so. In his youth, he had possessed a small plot of good land and dreams of prosperity. But the English landlords had taken the best fields for themselves, leaving the Irish tenants to scratch out a living on rocky soil that yielded little more than stones and sorrow. Each year brought new taxes, new demands, and new reasons for the English to squeeze what little remained from the Irish peasants. Seamus had watched his dreams crumble like the walls of his cottage, and with them had gone whatever kindness might have once lived in his heart.

He took his frustrations out on his children, but most especially on Mary. She was the easiest target, the smallest, the weakest, the one who could not fight back. When the crops failed, when the landlord came demanding rent, when the weight of his failures pressed too heavily upon his shoulders, Seamus would reach for his leather belt or his walking stick, and Mary would know to run. But there was nowhere to run in a one-room cottage, nowhere to hide from a man whose rage needed an outlet and who had long since stopped caring about the consequences of his actions.

The beatings began when Mary was barely old enough to walk. At first, they were sporadic moments of explosive anger that passed as quickly as they came. But as the years wore on and the family's circumstances grew more desperate, the violence became routine. Mary learned to read the signs: the way her father's jaw would tighten when he counted their meager stores of grain, the particular set of his shoulders when he returned from the village with news of another neighbor evicted from their land, the dangerous glint in his eyes when he had been drinking the harsh whiskey that burned away his sorrows and his conscience in equal measure.

By the time Mary was seven years old, her body was a map of bruises and scars. She had learned to move carefully, to speak softly, to make herself as small and invisible as possible. But invisibility was impossible in a space so cramped, and silence was no protection against a man who saw her very existence as an affront to his dignity and his dreams.

Her brothers, following their father's example, treated Mary with casual cruelty. They would trip her as she carried water from the well, push her face into the mud when she tried to eat, and steal what little food she managed to claim for herself. They called her names that cut deeper than any physical blow, bastard, curse, devil's spawn. They told her stories of changelings and demons, convincing her that she was not truly their sister but some evil thing left in place of the real child who had died with their mother.

Brigid was perhaps the cruellest of all, for she possessed the intelligence to make her torments more sophisticated and lasting. She would whisper to Mary in the dark of night, telling her that their mother's ghost walked the cottage, searching for the daughter who had killed her. She would hide Mary's few possessions, a rag doll made from scraps, a smooth stone she had found by the river, and then help their father search for them, suggesting that Mary had stolen food or money and hidden the evidence.

The village of Ballymore offered no refuge for a childlike Mary. The other families had their own struggles, their own mouths to feed, their own children to protect. They saw the Costello's as cursed, marked by tragedy and poverty in ways that might be contagious. The priest, Father O'Brien, was an old man more concerned with his own comfort than the welfare of his parishioners. When Mary appeared at church with fresh bruises, he would speak vaguely of God's plan and the importance of honouring one's father, but he never intervened, never offered sanctuary or even a kind word.

The women of the village whispered about Mary when they thought she could not hear. They spoke of the circumstances of her birth, of the way her mother had died cursing, of the strange accidents and misfortunes that seemed to follow the Costello family. Some said the child was marked by the devil, others that she carried her mother's angry spirit within her. All agreed that she was trouble, a dark presence that brought ill luck to anyone who showed her kindness.

As Mary grew older, the nature of the abuse she suffered began to change. Her father's violence became more calculated, more deliberately cruel. He would force her to kneel on sharp stones for hours as punishment for imagined transgressions. He would deny her food for days at a time, telling her that she had to earn her place at the table through perfect obedience and service. He would make her sleep outside in all weather, claiming that the cottage was too crowded and that she, being the least important member of the family, should be the one to sacrifice her comfort.

But it was not only her father whose treatment of Mary grew more sinister as she approached womanhood. Her brothers, now young men themselves, began to look at her with a different kind of hunger. They would corner her when their father was away, touching her in ways that made her skin crawl, making suggestions that filled her with a terror deeper than any beating. They spoke of her as if she were property, something to be used and discarded when they were tired of the game.

The worst of them was Padraig, the eldest, who had inherited their fathe''s capacity for cruelty but possessed none of his restraint. He would grab Mary when she was alone, pressing her against the stone walls of the cottage, his hands rough and demanding. He would whisper threats in her ear, promising that if she told anyone what he did, he would make sure she suffered in ways that would make their father's beatings seem like gentle caresses.

Mary learned to live in a state of constant vigilance, always watching, always listening, always ready to run or hide or fight if necessary. She developed an almost supernatural ability to sense danger, to read the moods and intentions of those around her. It was a skill that would serve her well in the years to come, though she could not have known it then.

The turning point came on a cold February morning when Mary was fourteen years old. She had been sent to the well to fetch water, a task that required her to walk nearly a mile from the cottage through fields still hard with frost. The bucket was heavy and the path treacherous, but she had made this journey countless times before. What she had not expected was to find Padraig waiting for her in the grove of oak trees that stood halfway between the cottage and the well.

He had been drinking, she could smell the whiskey on his breath from several feet away, and his eyes held a wildness that made her stomach clench with fear. He spoke to her in the crude language he had learned from the other young men in the village, telling her what he intended to do, how he had been watching her and waiting for the right moment. He said that she owed him this, that she owed all of them this, for the trouble she had brought to their family.

Mary tried to run, but Padraig was stronger and faster. He caught her easily, dragging her deeper into the grove where the trees would hide them from any passersby. She fought him with a desperation born of pure terror, clawing at his face, kicking at his shins, screaming for help that she knew would not come. But her struggles only seemed to excite him more, and when he finally pinned her to the frozen ground, she could see in his eyes that he meant to take from her the one thing she still possessed that was truly her own.

It was then that something changed in Mary Costello. Later, she would remember the moment with perfect clarity, the way the world seemed to slow and sharpen around her, the way her fear transformed into something harder and more dangerous. Her hand, scrabbling desperately in the dirt and dead leaves, closed around a stone the size of her fist. Without conscious thought, without hesitation, she brought it up with all her strength and struck Padraig in the temple.

The sound it made was unlike anything she had ever heard, a wet, hollow crack that seemed to echo through the grove long after the stone had fallen from her hand. Padraig's eyes went wide with surprise, then vacant, and he collapsed on top of her, his weight suddenly dead and crushing. Blood, dark and thick, began to pool beneath his head, staining the frost-covered earth.

Mary lay there for what felt like hours, trapped beneath her brother's body, feeling his blood seep through her clothes and onto her skin. She waited for him to move, to breathe, to curse her and strike her as he had done so many times before. But Padraig Costello would never move again, would never hurt her or anyone else, would never draw another breath in this world or any other.

When she finally managed to push his body aside and struggle to her feet, Mary felt something fundamental shift inside her. The fear that had been her constant companion for fourteen years was still there, but it was joined now by something else, 2a cold, calculating awareness of her own capacity for violence. She had killed a man, her own brother, and while part of her was horrified by what she had done, another part felt a satisfaction so deep and pure that it frightened her more than any beating ever had.

She looked down at Padraig's still form, at the blood that continued to spread across the ground, at the stone that lay beside his head like an accusation. She knew that she should feel remorse, should weep for the life she had taken, and should pray for forgiveness and mercy. Instead, she felt only a strange sense of completion, as if she had finally discovered her true nature after years of pretending to be something she was not.

The practical considerations came to her quickly. She could not leave Padraig's body here to be discovered, the consequences would be swift and terrible. Her father would kill her if the English authorities did not hang her first. She needed to hide what she had done, to make it appear as if her brother had met with some accident or simply disappeared.

With a strength she had not known she possessed, Mary dragged Padraig's body deeper into the grove, to a place where the trees grew thick and the undergrowth was dense. She covered him with branches and leaves, with stones and dirt, until no trace of him remained visible. She cleaned the blood from her clothes as best she could with handfuls of snow, and she threw the stone that had killed him into the deepest part of the nearby bog, where it would sink without a trace.

When she returned to the cottage hours later, carrying the water she had originally set out to fetch, her father demanded to know where she had been for so long. She told him that she had fallen through the ice at the well and had needed time to dry her clothes and warm herself. He struck her for her clumsiness, but it was a perfunctory blow, lacking the vicious intent of his usual punishments. He was more concerned with Padraig's absence, the young man had not returned from whatever errand had taken him from the cottage that morning.

For three days, the family searched for Padraig. They combed the fields and the village, questioned neighbours and strangers, and offered what little they could afford as a reward for information. Mary joined in the search with apparent concern, calling her brother's name and peering into ditches and abandoned buildings with the same desperate hope as the rest of them. She was careful to avoid the grove where his body lay hidden, but she felt his presence there like a weight on her conscience.

On the fourth day, they found traces of him—or rather, what the wild animals had left behind. A torn piece of his shirt caught on a thorn bush, some bones scattered by scavengers, enough to suggest that Padraig Costello had met with some terrible accident in the wilderness. The family mourned him as they had mourned their mother, with tears and prayers and bitter acceptance of their fate. Only Mary knew the truth, and she carried that knowledge like a secret flame burning in her chest.

The months that followed Padraig's disappearance brought unexpected changes to the Costello household. Without her eldest brother's cruel influence, the other boys seemed less inclined to torment Mary. Her father, grief-stricken by the loss of his firstborn son, paid little attention to any of his remaining children. For the first time in her life, Mary experienced something approaching peace.

But peace, she discovered, was not the same as happiness. The knowledge of what she had done, of what she was capable of doing, colored every moment of her existence. She found herself studying the faces of her family members, wondering what it would take to make them stop breathing, how easy it would be to arrange accidents for each of them in turn. The thoughts came unbidden and unwelcome, but they came nonetheless, and with each passing day, they seemed less shocking and more natural.

It was during this period of relative calm that Mary first began to see her brother's ghost. It started as glimpses from the corner of her eye, a familiar figure standing at the edge of the grove, a shadow that moved when no living thing was there to cast it. She told herself it was guilt, imagination, the product of a mind strained by secrets and lies. But as the weeks passed, the apparition became more solid, more persistent, and more undeniably real.

Padraig's ghost was not the vengeful spectre she might have expected. Instead, he appeared much as he had in life, but with a sadness that had never been there before. He would stand at the foot of her sleeping place in the cottage, watching her with eyes that held no anger, only a profound and terrible understanding. Sometimes he would mouth words she could not hear, gestures she could not interpret. Other times, he would simply stand there, a reminder of what she had done and what she had become.

Mary tried to ignore the ghost, to pretend that she could not see him, but Padraig's presence was as persistent in death as his cruelty had been in life. He followed her to the well, stood beside her as she worked in the fields, and sat across from her during the family's meagre meals. No one else seemed aware of him, and Mary began to wonder if she was losing her mind, if the weight of her secret was driving her to madness.

But madness, she realised, might be a mercy compared to the alternative. For as the months turned to years, and as Mary grew from a girl into a young woman, she began to understand that killing Padraig had not been an aberration, a moment of desperate self-defence that would never be repeated. Instead, it had been a revelation, an awakening to her true nature and her true purpose in this world.

The other members of her family began to seem less like people and more like problems to be solved. Her father's drunken rages, her remaining brothers' casual cruelties, her sister's poisonous tongue, all of these things could be ended with the right application of force at the right moment. The knowledge was intoxicating and terrifying in equal measure, a power that she had never imagined she could possess.

Mary Costello was seventeen years old when she killed for the second time, and by then she had learned to plan more carefully, to think beyond the immediate moment of violence to the consequences that would follow. Her victim was her brother Cormac, the second eldest, who had begun to display the same predatory interest in her that Padraig had shown. But this time, Mary was ready for him.

She lured him to the old stone bridge that crossed the stream at the edge of their property, telling him that she had found something there that he would want to see. It was a moonless night in late autumn, and the water below ran swift and deep with the recent rains. When Cormac leaned over the bridge's low wall to peer into the darkness below, Mary struck him with a piece of broken stone, sending him tumbling into the rushing water.

His body was found three days later, caught in the roots of a fallen tree nearly two miles downstream. The village constable declared it an accidental death, the bridge was known to be treacherous in the dark, and Cormac had been drinking heavily that evening. No one questioned Mary's story that she had been asleep in the cottage when her brother left for his fatal walk.

But Cormac's ghost joined Padraig's within a week of the funeral, and now Mary found herself accompanied by two silent, sorrowful spirits wherever she went. They stood together at the foot of her sleeping place, walked beside her through the fields, sat with her during the long, cold evenings when the wind howled around the cottage walls. Their presence was a constant reminder of what she had done and what she was becoming, but it was also, in a strange way, a comfort. They were hers now, bound to her by the violence that had ended their lives, and they would never leave her alone again.

The pattern was established now, and Mary found herself caught in its inexorable rhythm. Each death made the next one easier, more natural, more necessary. Her remaining brothers fell one by one, Seamus, the younger, to a fall from the cottage roof while making repairs, Brendan to a fever that might have been helped by medicine if Mary had not hidden the herbs that could have saved him. Each death brought another ghost to join her growing collection of silent companions.

Her sister Brigid proved more challenging, being naturally suspicious and possessed of a cunning that matched Mary's own. But even she could not escape the fate that Mary had planned for her. A contaminated well, a suggestion that the water tasted strange, a helpful offer to fetch fresh water from the stream, it was almost too easy. Brigid's death was attributed to the same fever that had claimed Brendan, and her ghost joined the others in their eternal vigil around Mary's sleeping place.

By the time Mary was twenty years old, she was alone in the cottage with her father, surrounded by the ghosts of her siblings and possessed of a reputation in the village as a young woman marked by tragedy. The neighbours whispered about the curse that seemed to follow the Costello family, about the way death stalked their household like a hungry wolf. Some of the older women crossed themselves when Mary passed, and mothers pulled their children closer when she walked through the village square.

Seamus Costello, broken by the loss of his children and aged beyond his years by grief and drink, barely seemed to notice that his daughter was the only one left. He spent his days staring into the fire, muttering prayers and curses in equal measure, drinking whatever whiskey he could afford and sleeping the sleep of the damned. He had become a shell of a man, hollowed out by loss and guilt and the terrible weight of his own failures.

Mary watched him with the same calculating gaze she had turned on her siblings, but she found herself reluctant to complete the work she had begun. Not out of any remaining affection, that had died long ago under the weight of his fists and his indifference, but because she was not yet ready to be entirely alone in the world. The ghosts were company of a sort, but they could not speak to her, could not answer her questions or share her burdens. Her father, broken as he was, remained her last connection to the world of the living.

But that connection, too, would eventually be severed. On a night in early spring, when the wind carried the scent of new growth and the promise of warmer days to come, Seamus Costello drank himself into a stupor deeper than any he had achieved before. Mary found him slumped over the table where he had been sitting, his breathing shallow and laboured, his skin grey and cold to the touch.

She could have helped him then. Could have turned him on his side so that he would not choke on his own vomit, could have covered him with blankets to keep him warm, could have fetched the priest or the doctor or any of the neighbours who might have been able to save him. Instead, she sat in her chair by the fire and watched him die, counting each rattling breath until there were no more to count.

Seamus Costello's ghost was different from those of his children. Where they appeared sad and resigned, he seemed angry, confused, as if he could not understand how he had come to this end. He would pace the cottage at night, his spirit feet making no sound on the dirt floor, his ghostly hands reaching for bottles that were no longer there. Sometimes he would stop in front of Mary and stare at her with eyes that held a terrible knowledge, as if he finally understood what she had become and what she had done to his family.

Mary was now entirely alone in the cottage, surrounded by the ghosts of her family and possessed of a reputation that made her both feared and pitied by the people of Ballymore. She was twenty-one years old, unmarried and unmarriageable, with no family to protect her and no prospects for the future. By all rights, she should have been destitute, dependent on the charity of the church or the grudging assistance of distant relatives.

But Mary Costello had learned to be resourceful in ways that would have shocked the good people of the village. The deaths of her family members had not been entirely without benefit, there were small inheritances, possessions that could be sold, debts that died with the debtors. More importantly, she had discovered that her reputation as a woman touched by tragedy could be turned to her advantage in unexpected ways.

The village had its share of people with problems that could not be solved through conventional means. Wives who wished to be widows, children who stood to inherit if only certain relatives would pass away, and merchants who found their competitors inconveniently successful. These people began to seek out Mary Costello, drawn by whispers and rumours, by the knowledge that death seemed to follow in her wake like a faithful hound.

They came to her cottage in the dark of night, speaking in hushed tones of their troubles and their desires. They paid her in coins and goods, in favours and information, in the currency of desperation and guilt. Mary listened to their requests with the same calm attention she had once given to her father's drunken ramblings, and she began to understand that she had found her calling, her purpose in a world that had never wanted her.

The first person she killed for money was the wife of a blacksmith in the neighbouring village of Drummore. The woman had been beating her children, starving them, selling their clothes and food to buy gin for herself. The blacksmith, a good man driven to desperation by his wife's cruelty, came to Mary with tears in his eyes and a purse full of silver coins. He did not ask her directly to kill his wife, such words were too dangerous to speak aloud, but his meaning was clear enough.

Mary accepted the commission with the same businesslike efficiency she had brought to the deaths of her own family. She studied the blacksmith's wife, learned her habits and weaknesses, and discovered that the woman had a fondness for a particular type of berry that grew wild in the hills. It was a simple matter to gather the berries, to treat them with certain herbs and powders that Mary had learned about from an old woman who lived alone in the bog, and to leave them where the blacksmith's wife would find them.

The woman died in agony three days later; her body wracked with convulsions and her mouth foaming with poison. The village doctor declared it a case of accidental poisoning, such things happened when people were careless about what they gathered from the wild. The blacksmith mourned his wife publicly and paid Mary the rest of her fee privately, and his children grew fat and happy under the care of the kind woman he married six months later.

The blacksmith's wife became the first ghost who was not a member of Mary's family, and her presence among the others marked a new chapter in Mary Costello's life. She was no longer simply a woman who had killed to survive or to escape abuse. She had become something else entirely, a death dealer solver of problems that could not be solved by law or custom or prayer.

Word of her services spread slowly but surely through the network of whispers and rumours that connected the villages and towns of rural Ireland. People began to seek her out from greater and greater distances, bringing their troubles and their coins, their desperate needs and their guilty consciences. Mary's cottage became a place of pilgrimage for those who had exhausted all other options, who had nowhere else to turn in their extremity.

She developed a reputation for discretion and efficiency, for deaths that appeared natural and investigations that led nowhere. She learned to read people with the same skill she had once used to anticipate her father's moods, to understand what they truly wanted even when they could not bring themselves to say it aloud. She became an expert in the use of poisons and accidents, in the timing of coincidences and the art of misdirection.

But with each death she arranged, each life she ended for coin and favour, Mary's collection of ghosts grew larger and more restless. They filled her cottage now, standing in every corner, sitting at her table, lying in her bed. They watched her with eyes that held no judgment but infinite sadness, as if they understood better than she did the price she was paying for her newfound prosperity.

The ghosts never spoke to her, never tried to prevent her from killing again, never offered warnings or advice. They simply existed, a constant reminder of the lives she had taken and the souls she had sent into whatever darkness awaited beyond the veil of death. Their presence was both comforting and terrifying, a sign that she was never truly alone but also never truly free from the consequences of her actions.

As Mary Costello entered her twenty-fifth year, she had become the most feared and sought-after woman in three counties, though few would have admitted to knowing her name or her business. She lived alone in her cottage with her ghosts, surrounded by the wealth she had accumulated through murder and the reputation she had built on the bones of her victims. She had found her place in the world at last, carved out a niche for herself through violence and cunning and the ruthless application of her particular talents.

But even as she counted her coins and planned her next killing, Mary could not escape the feeling that she was being watched by more than just the ghosts of her victims. There was something else in the shadows of her cottage, something that had been there since the night she killed Padraig in the grove of oak trees. It was patient and persistent, growing stronger with each life she took, feeding on the violence and death that had become the foundation of her existence.

Mary Costello had become a murderess, but she was beginning to suspect that she was not the only predator stalking the hills and villages of Ireland. Something else was hunting in the darkness, something that had been drawn to her by the scent of blood and the promise of more deaths to come. And as she sat in her cottage surrounded by the ghosts of her victims, Mary began to wonder if she had become the hunter or the hunted, the killer or the prey in a game whose rules she was only beginning to understand.

The weight of stones had shaped her from birth, had driven her to violence and murder and the accumulation of wealth built on death. But now, as she looked into the shadows where something waited and watched, Mary Costello began to suspect that the heaviest stone of all was yet to fall, and when it did, it would crush not just her victims but herself as well. The ghosts knew it too, shc could see it in their sad, knowing eyes, but like everything else in her life, this knowledge came too late to change the course she had set for herself so many years ago in a grove of oak trees with her brother's blood on her hands.

Chapter Two
The Watcher in the Bog

The thing that had been watching Mary Costello since her first kill had a name, though it had not spoken that name aloud in more than three centuries. It called itself An Dubhán, the Hook, and it was older than the stones that dotted the Irish countryside, older than the bog that stretched beyond Mary's cottage like a sea of black water and rotting vegetation.

An Dubhán had been born in the time before Christ walked the earth, when the Celts still offered blood sacrifices to gods whose names were forgotten even by the wind. It had fed then on the life force of warriors and druids, on the terror of those who died screaming in the sacred groves while their blood watered the roots of ancient oaks. But the old ways had faded, the old gods had turned their faces away, and An Dubhán had been forced to adapt or starve.

It had learned patience in the long centuries that followed. It had discovered that while the grand sacrifices of the past were gone, there was still plenty of death to be found among the common people, plague and famine, war and murder, the endless cycle of violence that seemed to be humanity's greatest gift to the world. An Dubhán had fed on all of it, growing stronger with each life that ended in fear and pain, each soul that departed this world carrying the weight of unfinished business.

But Mary Costello was different. In her, An Dubhán had found something it had not encountered for generations, a mortal who killed not out of desperation or madness or momentary rage, but with the cold calculation of a predator. She was an artist of death, a craftsman of murder, and watching her work was like witnessing the birth of something magnificent and terrible.

From the shadows of the bog, An Dubhán had observed every killing, had tasted the fear of each victim, had savoured the moment when life fled from their eyes. It had grown fat on the deaths Mary arranged, had felt its power swell with each new ghost that joined the growing congregation in her cottage. She was feeding it in ways she could not possibly understand, nurturing it with a feast of violence that had awakened hungers An Dubhán had almost forgotten it possessed.

But now, as it watched her count the coins from her latest commission, An Dubhán felt something else stirring in the ancient depths of its consciousness, a recognition, a kinship, a desire that transcended mere feeding. Mary Costello was not just another mortal to be used and discarded. She was something rarer and more precious: a worthy partner, a kindred spirit, a creature who understood the true nature of power in this world.

The time had come, An Dubhán decided, to make itself known.

The first sign that something had changed came on a Tuesday morning in late October, when Mary woke to find that all of her ghosts had vanished.

She sat up in her narrow bed, scanning the cottage with eyes that had grown accustomed to the constant presence of her spectral companions. The corner where her father usually paced was empty. The space beside the hearth where Padraig and Cormac typically stood was vacant. Even the blacksmith's wife, who had taken to sitting at the table where she had once counted her gin money, was nowhere to be seen.

The silence in the cottage was profound and unsettling. For years, Mary had lived with the whisper of ghostly movement, the barely perceptible shift of air that marked their passage through her small world. Without them, the space felt hollow, echoing, as if the very walls had been stripped of some essential presence that had given them meaning.

Mary dressed quickly and stepped outside, hoping to catch a glimpse of her departed spirits in the morning mist. The bog stretched before her, its surface dark as ink beneath a grey sky that promised rain. The wind carried the familiar scents of peat and decay, of water that had stood stagnant for a thousand years, of things that had died and been forgotten in the depths of the earth.

But there was something else in the air now, a presence that made the hair on her arms stand upright, that set her teeth on edge like the taste of copper pennies. Something was watching her from the bog, something that did not belong to the world of the living or the recently dead.

"Mary Costello."

The voice came from everywhere and nowhere, seeming to rise from the very ground beneath her feet. It was neither male nor female, neither young nor old, but something that existed beyond such mortal distinctions. It spoke her name with the familiarity of an old friend and the authority of a judge pronouncing sentence.

Mary's hand moved instinctively to the kitchen knife she kept tucked in her belt, a habit born of years spent among people who might wish her harm. But even as her fingers closed around the handle, she understood that steel would be useless against whatever had spoken her name.

"Who are you?" she called out, her voice steady despite the fear that clawed at her throat. "What do you want?"

The laughter that answered her was like the sound of autumn leaves rustling in a dead tree, like the whisper of wind through empty graves. It seemed to come from the bog itself, as if the very landscape were amused by her question.

"I am the hunger that follows in your wake," the voice replied. "I am the shadow that feeds on the fear of your victims. I am the one who has been watching you, learning from you, growing strong on the deaths you so artfully arrange."

A figure began to materialise at the edge of the bog, rising from the dark water like something born from a nightmare. It was tall and gaunt, wrapped in shadows that seemed to move independently of any earthly wind. Its face was a void where features should have been, a darkness so complete that looking at it made Mary's eyes water and her head spin.

"You have been feeding me for years without knowing it." An Dubhán continued, its voice now seeming to come from the figure itself. "Every life you take, every death you orchestrate, every moment of terror you create, all of it nourishes me, sustains me, makes me stronger than I have been in centuries""

Mary felt her knees grow weak, but she forced herself to remain standing. She had faced death before, had looked into the eyes of her victims as life fled from them, but this was different. This was something that existed outside the natural order, something that predated human understanding of what was possible in the world.

"Are you... Are you the devil?" she whispered, the words dragging themselves from her throat like broken glass.

The figure tilted its head, and Mary thought she could see something that might have been amusement in the depths of its featureless face.

"I am older than your devil, child. I walked this land when your god was still a story whispered around campfires, when the people who lived here offered blood to forces that your priests cannot even name. I am what remains when all other gods have been forgotten, hunger itself, given form and purpose."

An Dubhán began to move closer, its feet seeming to glide over the surface of the bog water without causing so much as a ripple. As it approached, Mary could feel the temperature around her dropping, could see her breath beginning to mist in the suddenly frigid air.

"But I did not come here to frighten you, Mary Costello. I came to make you an offer."

The creature stopped just beyond arm's reach, and Mary could now see that what she had taken for a face was actually a swirling vortex of shadow and starlight, a window into someplace that existed far beyond the boundaries of the mortal world. Looking into it was like staring into the space between the stars, into the cold emptiness that lay at the heart of all things.

"You have a gift," An Dubhán said, its voice now soft and almost seductive. "A talent for death that is rare among mortals. But you are limited by your humanity, constrained by the weaknesses of flesh and blood. You grow tired, you make mistakes, you leave evidence that clever men might eventually uncover."

Mary found her voice at last, though it came out as barely more than a croak. "What are you offering me?"

"Partnership," the creature replied. "Power beyond anything you have ever imagined. I can teach you methods of killing that will leave no trace, no ghost, no lingering evidence of your involvement. I can show you how to strike from a distance, how to arrange deaths that will appear so natural that even the most suspicious observer will find nothing to question."

The offer hung in the air between them like a serpent coiled to strike. Mary could feel the weight of it, the magnitude of what was being proposed. This creature, this thing that called itself older than devils, was offering to make her into something more than human, something more deadly and efficient than she had ever dreamed of becoming.

"And in return?" she asked, though she suspected she already knew the answer.

"In return, you will feed me as you have been doing, but more deliberately, more abundantly. I will guide you to prey that will satisfy both our appetites, the wealthy, the powerful, those whose deaths will cause ripples that spread far beyond the boundaries of these small villages. Together, we will feast on fear and death and the delicious terror of those who believe themselves safe from harm."

Mary closed her eyes, feeling the weight of the decision pressing down on her like a stone. She thought of her cottage filled with ghosts, of the coins hidden beneath her floorboards, of the reputation that had made her both feared and sought after throughout the countryside. She had built a life for herself through murder and cunning, had carved out a place in the world through violence and careful planning.

But this creature was offering her more than just continued survival. It was offering her transcendence, elevation beyond the limitations that had always constrained her. She could become something legendary, something that would be whispered about in fearful tones long after her mortal body had crumbled to dust.

When she opened her eyes, An Dubhán was watching her with what she somehow knew was infinite patience. It had waited centuries for this moment, had fed on lesser prey while searching for someone worthy of its partnership. It could wait a little longer for her answer.

"My ghosts," Mary said finally. "Where are they?"

"Dismissed," An Dubhán replied. "You will have no need of such reminders once you accept my offer. The dead will trouble you no more, for you will be serving purposes far grander than their petty concerns with justice or revenge."

Mary looked back at her cottage, at the simple stone walls that had sheltered her through years of killing and accumulation. It seemed suddenly small and shabby, a peasant's hovel that was beneath the dignity of what she might become. She could feel the creature's power radiating from its shadowy form, could sense the vast knowledge and ancient hunger that dwelt within it.

"Yes," she said, the word escaping her lips before she had fully decided to speak it. "Yes, I accept your offer."

An Dubhán's form seemed to pulse with satisfaction, and the temperature around them dropped even further. Mary's breath came out in great white clouds now, and frost began to form on the grass at her feet.

"Then let us begin your education, Mary Costello. There is much you must learn, and the night is still young."

The creature extended what might have been a hand toward her, though it was difficult to tell where the shadows ended and its actual form began. Mary reached out without hesitation, and when her fingers touched the writhing darkness, she felt a cold so intense that it burned, a sensation like touching the surface of a frozen star.

Images flooded her mind, visions of deaths she had never imagined, techniques of murder that transcended anything she had learned through trial and error. She saw ways to kill from great distances, methods of poison that would leave no trace in the victim's body, accidents so perfectly arranged that they would defy all investigation. She saw herself moving through the world like a force of nature, striking down targets with the precision of lightning and the inevitability of winter.

But more than that, she saw what she could become. The creature showed her visions of herself decades hence, no longer confined to her simple cottage but moving through the grand houses of the wealthy and powerful. She saw herself as a lady of substance and influence, feared and respected by those who mattered, her reputation built not on whispered rumours but on undeniable results.

When the visions ended, and Mary found herself once again standing beside the bog, she was no longer the same woman who had woken that morning to find her ghosts missing. Something fundamental had changed within her, some essential boundary had been crossed. She could feel An Dubhán's presence nestled in her mind now, not controlling her thoughts but sharing them, offering guidance and knowledge as she needed it.

"Our first target," the creature whispered in her mind, "lives in a great house twenty miles to the south. He is a magistrate who has grown rich through corruption and cruelty, who has sentenced innocent men to death while allowing the guilty to purchase their freedom. His death will serve justice while providing us with both profitand nourishment."

Mary smiled, and for the first time in her life, the expression held no trace of the fear or desperation that had always lurked beneath her careful composure. She was no longer a peasant girl who killed to survive or a village witch who murdered for coins. She was something new, something unprecedented in the history of the world, a mortal woman armed with the knowledge of an ancient god of death.

“Tell me about him,” she said aloud, her voice carrying easily across the still water of the bog.“Tell me everything I need to know.”

An Dubhán's laughter rippled through the air around them, and somewhere in the distance, a murder of crows took flight from the dead trees that marked the bog's far edge. The sound of their wings was like applause, like celebration, like the rustle of dark curtains being drawn across the stage where Mary Costello would perform the greatest role of her life.

The partnership had begun, and the world would never be the same.

Chapter Three
The Magistrate's End

The house of Magistrate Cornelius Blackwood stood on a hill overlooking the River Nore, its Georgian facade gleaming white against the dark Irish sky like the bones of some massive creature picked clean by carrion birds. It was a monument to English wealth and Irish suffering, built with stone quarried by hands that would never be permitted to cross its threshold, furnished with luxuries purchased with the blood and tears of those who appeared before its master's bench.

Mary Costello crouched in the shadow of an ancient yew tree at the edge of the estate grounds, studying the house with eyes that had learned to see patterns invisible to ordinary mortals. For three days, she had watched the comings and goings of the household, memorising the routines of servants and the habits of their master. An Dubhán whispered constantly in her mind now, pointing out details she might have missed, suggesting approaches she would never have considered on her own.

"The kitchen maid," the creature murmured in her thoughts, its voice like silk drawn across a blade. "She arrives before dawn and leaves after sunset. Tired, overworked, and paid barely enough to keep body and soul together. She would be grateful for a few extra coins, and she asks no questions about their source."

Mary nodded almost imperceptibly. She had identified the girl herself, a wan, hollow-cheeked creature of perhaps sixteen years who moved through the kitchen gardens like a ghost, gathering herbs and vegetables for the magistrate's table. Her name was Bridget Murphy, and she had the look of someone who had learned early that survival depended on invisibility and silence.

"And the magistrate himself?" Mary whispered, though she knew An Dubhán could hear her thoughts as clearly as her spoken words.

"Creatures of habit are the easiest prey," came the reply. "Every morning at precisely nine o'clock, he takes his breakfast in the conservatory overlooking the river. Porridge with cream, two eggs prepared precisely to his liking, tea so hot it steams his spectacles. He reads the Cork Examiner while he eats, and he allows no interruptions during this sacred ritual."

Mary smiled in the darkness. She had observed this routine herself, had watched through the tall windows as the magistrate performed his morning ceremony with the punctuality of a church bell. Cornelius Blackwood was a man who believed that order and routine were the foundations of civilisation, who structured his days according to principles of English efficiency and Protestant virtue. He would never suspect that his very predictability would be the instrument of his destruction.

"The method?" she asked, though she suspected she already knew what An Dubhán would suggest.

"Digitalis," the creature replied with something that might have been amusement. "The foxglove that grows so abundantly in these Irish hills. A few leaves steeped in his morning tea, and his heart will stop within the hour. To all observers, it will appear that Magistrate Blackwood has suffered a natural death, tragic, perhaps, but hardly suspicious for a man of his age and temperament."

Mary had already gathered the foxglove, had prepared the extract using knowledge that An Dubhán had poured directly into her mind during their first night together. The poison was odourless and nearly tasteless, and it would leave no trace that any physician in Ireland would know how to detect. More importantly, it would cause the kind of death that powerful men feared most, sudden, undignified, and utterly beyond their control.

The kitchen maid appeared at the servants' entrance just as the church bells of the distant village chimed five o'clock. Mary watched as the girl lit a candle and made her way through the darkened house to begin her day's labours. In an hour, she would begin preparing the magistrate's breakfast, and in that hour, Mary Costello would transform from observer to participant in the ancient dance of death.

Moving like a shadow across the estate grounds, Mary approached the servants' entrance with the confidence of someone who belonged there. She had dressed carefully for this morning's work, her clothes were clean but worn, her hair pinned back beneath a simple cap, her manner that of a woman seeking employment rather than planning murder. When she knocked softly on the kitchen door, it was with the hesitant rap of someone hoping for charity rather than the bold demand of an intruder.

Bridget Murphy opened the door with the wariness of someone who had learned that unexpected visitors rarely brought good news. But when she saw Mary, a woman not much older than herself, plainly dressed and carrying a small bundle that suggested a traveller seeking work, her expression softened slightly.

“We’re not hiring,” she said automatically, though her voice held more sympathy than dismissal. “The master’s very particular about the staff, and he doesn’t like changes to his routine.”

“I’m not looking for permanent employment,,” Mary replied, allowing just a touch of desperation to color her voice. “Just a day’s work, perhaps. I’ve been walking since before dawn, and I’ve had nothing to eat since yesterday morning. I can cook, clean, mend, whatever needs doing.”

The kitchen maid glanced nervously over her shoulder, then stepped aside to let Mary enter. The kitchen was warm and bright, already filled with the smells of bread baking and coffee brewing. It was the kind of kitchen that Mary had dreamed of as a child, spacious, well-appointed, stocked with ingredients that most Irish families would consider luxuries beyond imagining.

“I shouldn’t,” Bridget whispered, clearly torn between compassion and fear of her employer’s wrath. “If the master found out I let a stranger into his house...”

“He won’t find out,” Mary said gently, setting her bundle on a wooden table near the window. “I’ll help you with your morning tasks, take a bit of food for the road, and be gone before anyone knows I was here. What harm could there be in that?"

As she spoke, Mary let her hand rest casually on her bundle, feeling the small glass vial hidden within its folds.

The foxglove extract was ready, waiting only for the right moment to complete its deadly purpose. All she needed was access to the magistrate's morning tea, and the sympathetic kitchen maid would provide that access without ever knowing she had become an accomplice to murder.

"Well," Bridget said finally, glancing toward the stairs that led to the upper floors of the house. "I suppose you could help me prepare the master's breakfast. He's very particular about how things are done, but if you're careful...""I'm always careful," Mary replied, and meant it in ways the kitchen maid could never understand.

For the next hour, Mary worked alongside Bridget Murphy, learning the precise requirements of Magistrate Blackwood's morning meal. The porridge had to be stirred clockwise exactly forty-seven times. The eggs had to be turned at precisely the moment the whites began to set. The tea had to steep for exactly three minutes and thirty seconds, no more and no less.

It was during the preparation of the tea that Mary found her opportunity. While Bridget was occupied with the eggs, Mary carefully added three drops of the foxglove extract to the magistrate's teapot, watching as the colourless liquid disappeared into the dark brew without a trace. The deed was done so quickly and quietly that even An Dubhán, whispering approval in her mind, seemed impressed by her deftness.

"Perfect," the creature murmured as Mary resumed her tasks as if nothing had happened. "Now we wait for the morning''s entertainment to begin."

At precisely nine o'clock, the magistrate's breakfast was carried to the conservatory on a silver tray polished to mirror brightness. Mary watched from the kitchen doorway as Bridget arranged the meal with the precision of a religious ritual, placing each item in its designated location according to rules that had been established through years of repetition.

Magistrate Blackwood entered the conservatory like an actor taking his position on a familiar stage. He was a large man in his fifties, with the florid complexion and prominent belly of someone who had never known hunger or want. His clothes were of the finest English wool, his boots polished to perfection, his manner that of a man who had never doubted his right to command and be obeyed.

Mary retreated deeper into the kitchen as the magistrate seated himself at his table, but she maintained a clear view of the conservatory through the serving window. She watched as he unfolded his newspaper with practised efficiency, as he spooned his porridge with the mechanical precision of a clockwork figure, as he reached for his teacup with the confidence of a man performing a routine that had never varied in twenty years.

The first sip of tea passed without incident. So did the second and the third. Mary felt a moment of doubt, had she added too little of the extract? Had the foxglove lost its potency in the days since she had prepared it? But An Dubhán's presence in her mind remained calm and patient, radiating the confidence of something that had orchestrated death for millennia.

"Patience," the creature whispered. "The heart is a stubborn muscle, but it cannot resist forever. Watch, and learn how power dies."

It began as a slight tremor in the magistrate's left hand, barely noticeable as he turned the pages of his newspaper. Then came a tightness in his chest that made him pause in his reading, touching his sternum with the puzzled expression of someone experiencing an unfamiliar sensation. His breathing grew shallow and rapid, and a fine sheen of perspiration appeared on his forehead despite the cool morning air.

Magistrate Blackwood set down his teacup with hands that had begun to shake visibly. He tried to stand, perhaps intending to call for help, but his legs would no longer support him. He collapsed back into his chair with a sound that was part gasp and part moan, his face flushing red, then pale, then an alarming shade of blue.

The newspaper slipped from his nerveless fingers and scattered across the floor. His eyes, wide with the terror of a man who finally understood that his wealth and position could not protect him from the democracy of death, searched desperately for assistance that would not come. He tried to call out, but his voice emerged as nothing more than a hoarse whisper, a plea that dissolved into the morning air like mist.

Mary watched it all with the clinical detachment of a natural philosopher observing an interesting experiment. She noted the progression of symptoms, the exact timing of each stage, and the way the magistrate's body betrayed him in its final moments. This was education of the highest order, knowledge that could not be gained from books or conversation but only through direct observation of death in its most intimate moments.

Cornelius Blackwood died as the church bells chimed the half-hour, slumping forward in his chair with his face in what remained of his breakfast porridge. His final expression was one of profound surprise, as if he could not quite believe that the natural order of things, the order that had always placed him above the common run of humanity, had been so completely and suddenly overturned.

From the kitchen came the sound of Bridget Murphy calling for the magistrate, wondering why he had not rung for the breakfast tray to be cleared as was his custom. Mary listened as the girl's calls grew more urgent, as footsteps hurried through the house, as the terrible discovery was finally made.

The screaming began a moment later, not just from Bridget, but from the other servants who came running at the sound of her distress. Mary used the chaos as cover for her departure, slipping out the servants' entrance and into the estate grounds as the household erupted in panic and confusion behind her.

She walked calmly toward the road that would take her back to her cottage, her bundle once again slung over her shoulder, her manner that of someone who had completed a satisfactory morning's work. Behind her, she could hear the magistrate's coachman galloping toward the village to fetch the doctor, though they both knew it was far too late for medical intervention.

"Beautifully executed," An Dubhán purred in her mind as she put distance between herself and the scene of her latest crime. "Clean, efficient, and utterly beyond suspicion. The physician will declare it a natural death,, the heart failure that claims so many men of his age and habits. No one will think to look for poison, and even if they did, they would find no trace of it."

Mary smiled as she walked, feeling the familiar satisfaction that came with a job well done. But there was something else now, something deeper and more intoxicating than mere professional pride. She could feel An Dubhán's approval flowing through her like warm wine, could sense the creature's ancient hunger being sated by the fear and suffering it had witnessed through her eyes.

"And the payment?" she asked, though she already knew the answer.

"Hidden in a dead oak tree three miles south of the magistrate's estate," the creature replied. "Fifty gold sovereigns, as promised by our intermediary. Enough to live comfortably for months, or to purchase the materials and information needed for even more ambitious projects."

Mary nodded, already planning how she would retrieve the payment and what her next steps might be. The magistrate's death would cause ripples throughout the county, investigations, inquiries, perhaps even suspicions that his demise had been less than natural. But those ripples would eventually settle, and when they did, there would be other targets, other opportunities, other chances to demonstrate the deadly partnership she had formed with the ancient thing that whispered in her mind.

As she walked through the Irish countryside, Mary Costello no longer felt like a peasant girl who had stumbled into a trade she barely understood. She felt like what she had truly become, a force of nature disguised in human form, a bringer of death who moved through the world with purpose and precision that few mortals could comprehend.

The weight of stones had shaped her childhood, but now she carried a different kind of weight, the weight of knowledge, of power, of partnership with something that transcended mortal understanding. And unlike the stones that had once threatened to crush her, this new weight felt like wings.

Behind her, smoke began to rise from the direction of the magistrate's house as news of his sudden death spread through the estate and beyond. But Mary Costello did not look back. She had work to do, payments to collect, and a reputation to build that would make her the most feared and sought-after woman in all of Ireland.

The education An Dubhán had promised was only just beginning.

Chapter Four
The Taste of Gold

The gold sovereigns felt warm against Mary's palm, though they had been hidden in the hollow of the dead oak for three days before her arrival. Each coin bore the profile of King George IV, his stern features rendered in precious metal that represented more wealth than most Irish families would see in a lifetime. Fifty pieces of English gold, earned through the application of Irish cunning and ancient knowledge, it was a poetic justice that would have amused Mary if she had been given to such philosophical reflections.

But Mary Costello had little time for poetry. As she counted the coins in the fading light of evening, her mind was already turning toward practical matters. The magistrate's death had been clean and profitable, but it was only the beginning of what An Dubhán had promised her. The creature had spoken of greater targets, more ambitious schemes, deaths that would reshape the very balance of power in this corner of Ireland.

"You are pleased with your payment," An Dubhán observed, its voice carrying a note of something that might have been satisfaction. The creature's presence in her mind had grown stronger since their first collaboration, more intimate, more insistent. Sometimes Mary could feel it stirring in her thoughts like a cat settling in for a long sleep.

"I am pleased with the work," Mary replied, slipping the coins into a leather pouch that she tucked inside her bodice. "The magistrate died exactly as you predicted, and no one suspects anything more than natural causes. But this is just gold, and gold spends the same whether it comes from murder or honest labour."

"Ah, but this is not just gold," the creature corrected her, and Mary could sense its ancient amusement at her mortal perspective. "This is proof. Evidence that you can move among the powerful and wealthy, that you can strike at targets who believe themselves untouchable, that you can command payment worthy of your skills. Word of the magistrate's convenient demise will spread through certain circles, and with it will come offers of employment that dwarf what you earned in your cottage with your crude village poisons."

Mary felt a stirring of interest despite herself. She had grown comfortable with her reputation as a solver of domestic problems, the village witch who could arrange the death of an inconvenient spouse or troublesome relative. But An Dubhán was offering her something grander, more sophisticated, more in keeping with the education it had promised her.

"What kind of offers?" she asked, settling herself against the trunk of the dead oak as darkness gathered around them.

"There is a gathering, An Dubhán said, its voice dropping to barely more than a whisper in her mind. "Three days hence, in the port city of Cork; men of wealth and influence, English and Irish both, who have...

Difficulties that require delicate resolution. They meet in the back room of a tavern called The Merchant's Rest, ostensibly to discuss shipping investments and trade opportunities. But their true business is of a darker nature."Mary had heard whispers of such gatherings, shadowy assemblies where the powerful came to arrange the deaths of their rivals, the elimination of inconvenient witnesses, the removal of obstacles that stood between them and greater fortune. She had always dismissed such stories as tavern gossip, the fantasies of common people who needed to believe that the rich and mighty were as petty and murderous as anyone else.

"You want me to go to this meeting," she said, though it was not really a question.

"I want you to announce your availability," An Dubhán replied. "The magistrate's death will serve as your credentials, proof that you can deliver the kind of service they require. But you must be careful in how you present yourself. These are not desperate peasants seeking revenge on cruel landlords. These are sophisticated men who value discretion above all else, who will pay handsomely for results but who will kill without hesitation anyone who threatens their security."

The thought of walking into a room full of wealthy conspirators should have terrified Mary, but instead she felt a familiar thrill of anticipation. This was the next step in her evolution from village poisoner to something far more dangerous and lucrative. An Dubhán was offering her entry into a world she had never dreamed of accessing, where the stakes were higher but so were the rewards.

"How do I gain entry to such a gathering?" she asked. "They wont simply admit a stranger off the street."

"You will not go as Mary Costello, Irish peasant and suspected witch," the creature explained. "You will go as Mrs Catherine Blackthorne, recently widowed gentlewoman with connections to certain shipping interests in Liverpool. I will provide you with the necessary papers, the appropriate wardrobe, and the kind of refined speech that will convince them you belong in their company."

Mary blinked in surprise. The idea of transforming herself so completely, of stepping into an entirely different identity, was both thrilling and terrifying. She had learned to read and write from the old priest before he died, and she could speak properly when she chose to, but could she truly pass herself off as a lady of quality?

"The transformation will be more than mere costume and accent," An Dubhán continued, apparently reading her doubts. "I will share with you memories of the genteel life, knowledge of proper etiquette and social graces, familiarity with the world of commerce and politics that these men inhabit. When you enter that tavern, you will not be pretending to be Mrs Blackthorne, you will be her, completely and convincingly."

The prospect was intoxicating. Mary closed her eyes and tried to imagine herself dressed in silk and lace, speaking with the refined accent of the English gentry, moving through rooms filled with crystal and candlelight as if she had been born to such luxury. It seemed impossible, like a fairy tale told to comfort children who would never escape their humble circumstances.

But then again, three months ago, it would have seemed impossible that she would be sitting beneath a dead oak tree, counting gold earned through the murder of a magistrate, while conversing with an ancient creature of Irish legend. Impossibility, she was learning, was merely another word for opportunity that required courage to seize.

"When do we begin?" she asked.

The transformation took place over the next two days in Mary's cottage, though the simple stone building seemed to expand and reshape itself to accommodate what was happening within its walls. An Dubhán worked on Mary like a sculptor working clay, reshaping not just her appearance but her very essence, her understanding of herself and her place in the world.

The first change was physical. The creature's power flowed through Mary like ice-cold fire, straightening her posture, refining her features, smoothing away the calluses and scars that marked her as a woman who had known hard labour and harder treatment. Her hair, once lank and dull, became lustrous and manageable. Her skin, weathered by sun and wind, grew pale and smooth. Even her hands, marked by years of kitchen work and violence, became soft and elegant.

But the bigger changes were mental and emotional. An Dubhán poured knowledge into Mary's mind like wine into a cup, memories of drawing rooms and dinner parties, of conversations about politics and literature, of the subtle social codes that governed the behaviour of the English upper classes. She learned to walk differently, to hold her head at the proper angle, to speak with the precise diction that marked a woman of breeding and education.

More than that, she learned to think differently. The crude directness that had served her as a village poisoner was replaced by the sophisticated indirection prized by the wealthy and powerful. She learned to speak in implications and suggestions, to communicate deadly intentions through polite euphemisms, to negotiate murder as if it were merely another business transaction.

By the morning of the third day, Mary Costello had ceased to exist. In her place stood Mrs Catherine Blackthorne, a woman of obvious refinement and mysterious connections, dressed in a travelling costume of deep blue wool that had somehow appeared in the cottage overnight. Her luggage, leather cases of the finest quality, contained everything a genteel widow might need for a brief sojourn in Cork, clothes appropriate for any social occasion, jewellery that suggested wealth without ostentation, and papers documenting her identity and financial circumstances.

"Perfect," An Dubhán whispered as Mary examined herself in a mirror that had not been in the cottage the day before. "You are no longer the peasant girl who killed her brothers in fits of rage. You are a lady of quality who arranges deaths with the same care that others might arrange dinner parties."

Mary, Catherine, smiled at her reflection, and the expression was utterly different from any smile that had ever crossed Mary Costello's face. This was the smile of a woman who had never known hunger or fear, who had never been beaten or abused, who had been raised from birth to believe that the world existed for her convenience and pleasure.

"The coach will arrive within the hour," An Dubhán continued. "You will travel to Cork in comfort and style, as befits your station. The driver has been... Persuaded... to ask no questions about his passenger or her destination. When you arrive at The Merchant's Rest, you will be expected."

Catherine nodded, adjusting her gloves with practised elegance. She felt no trace of nervousness about the journey ahead, no doubt about her ability to move convincingly through the world of the wealthy and powerful. An Dubhán's transformation had been complete, she was no longer pretending to be someone else, she had become someone else entirely.

The coach that arrived was as elegant as everything else about her new identity, black lacquer and brass fittings, pulled by a matched pair of horses that would not have been out of place in the finest stables of England. The driver, a thin man with hollow eyes that suggested he had experienced An Dubhán's persuasion firsthand, helped her into the velvet-lined interior without speaking.

As Cork grew larger on the horizon, Catherine allowed herself a moment to appreciate the irony of her situation. She was travelling toward a gathering of conspirators and murderers while dressed as a lady of impeccable respectability, carrying credentials that would have opened doors in London or Dublin, transformed by an ancient Irish god into something that could move seamlessly through English society.

It was, she reflected, exactly the kind of revenge that her ancestors would have appreciated, the conquered becoming the conqueror, not through war or rebellion but through the simple expedient of becoming indistinguishable from their oppressors until the moment they chose to strike.

The Merchant's Rest proved to be exactly what she had expected, a tavern that catered to men of substance and discretion, with private rooms for sensitive conversations and staff who had learned the value of selective blindness and deafness. Catherine entered through the main door like any respectable lady seeking accommodation, her manner suggesting someone accustomed to the finest treatment wherever she went.

The landlord, a prosperous-looking man with the soft hands of someone who counted money rather than earning it through labour, greeted her with the deference due to her apparent station. When she mentioned that she had business with certain gentlemen who met privately to discuss commercial opportunities, his expression grew carefully neutral.

"Ah, yes, madam," he said, his voice carrying the studied discretion of someone who had hosted many such meetings. "The gentlemen you seek are expecting you, I believe. If you would be so kind as to follow me."

He led her through a maze of corridors to a heavy oak door set with iron hinges that suggested it had been built to keep secrets as well as intruders. The landlord knocked once, received a muffled response, and opened the door just wide enough for Catherine to enter.

The room beyond was thick with pipe smoke and the scent of expensive brandy. Six men sat around a table covered in green baize, their faces illuminated by the flickering light of oil lamps. They were all well-dressed, all middle-aged, all possessed of the kind of soft prosperity that came from years of successful exploitation of others' labor and desperation.

"Gentlemen," the landlord announced, "Mrs.

. Blackthorne has arrived."

Catherine stepped into the room with the confidence of a woman entering her own drawing room, sweeping the assembled company with a gaze that was both appraising and dismissive. These were wealthy men, powerful men, men accustomed to deference and obedience from their social inferiors. But as she studied their faces in the lamplight, Catherine could see the fear that lurked beneath their masks of respectability, the constant terror of losing what they had gained, of being exposed for what they truly were, of discovering that their wealth and position could not protect them from the democracy of death.

"Good evening, gentlemen," she said, her voice carrying the precise diction that An Dubhán had taught her. "I understand you have some business propositions that might interest a woman of my... Particular talents."

The silence that followed was pregnant with possibility and danger. Catherine could feel the weight of their collective gaze, the careful evaluation of men who had learned to judge people as potential assets or liabilities. But she also felt something else, the stirring of An Dubhán's hunger, the creature's anticipation as it prepared to feast on whatever violence and terror this meeting would produce.

One of the men, distinguished by a silver beard and clothes that spoke of London tailoring, finally spoke.

"We have heard of your recent work, Mrs Blackthorne," he said carefully. "The sudden demise of Magistrate Blackwood was... Most convenient for certain interests. We find ourselves hoping that such convenience might be available for other, similar situations."

Catherine smiled, and in that smile was all the deadly promise that had made Mary Costello the most feared woman in three counties. But now that promise wore silk gloves and spoke with a cultivated accent, and that made it infinitely more dangerous than it had ever been before.

"Gentlemen," she said, settling herself into the chair they indicated with practised grace, "I believe we have a great deal to discuss.""

Outside The Merchant's Rest, the fog was rolling in from Cork Harbour, wrapping the city in grey mist that muffled sound and obscured vision. It was perfect weather for the kind of business that would be conducted in that smoke-filled room, perfect conditions for the birth of conspiracies that would reshape the balance of power throughout Ireland.

And in the depths of that fog, something ancient and hungry stirred with anticipation, knowing that the feast it had been promised was about to begin in earnest.

Chapter Five
The Season of Blood

The contracts came faster than Catherine Blackthorne could have imagined. Within a fortnight of that first meeting at The Merchant's Rest, she found herself with a ledger full of names, each one representing a life to be ended and a purse to be filled. The gentlemen of Cork had been impressed by her refinement, her discretion, and most of all by the clean efficiency with which Magistrate Blackwood had been removed from the world. Word spread through the shadowy networks that connected the wealthy and powerful, and soon Catherine was receiving invitations to similar gatherings in Dublin, Belfast, and even London.

An Dubhán revelled in the abundance. The creature's presence in her mind had grown stronger with each successful kill, more substantial, more demanding. It fed not just on the deaths themselves but on the fear that preceded them, the terror of men and women who suddenly discovered that their wealth and position could not protect them from a force they never saw coming.

"You have become magnificent," the creature whispered as Catherine sat in the finest hotel room in Dublin, counting the gold that represented her latest commission.

"A dealer in death who moves through the highest circles of society like a serpent through Eden. They invite you to their tables, confide their secrets to you, and never suspect that they are entertaining their own destruction."

Catherine smiled as she arranged the coins into neat stacks. The transformation from Mary Costello to Catherine Blackthorne had been so complete that sometimes she forgot she had ever been anything else. The memories of her childhood in that squalid cottage felt like stories someone had told her about another person entirely. She had been reborn in silk and sophistication, baptised in the blood of her enemies, confirmed in a faith that recognised only power and the will to use it.

The first target after Cork had been Lord Pemberton, an English aristocrat who owned vast estates in County Kerry and was known for his particular cruelty toward his Irish tenants. His own nephew had approached Catherine at a soirée in Dublin, speaking in careful euphemisms about the difficulty of inheriting property when the current owner seemed determined to live forever. The young man had offered five hundred pounds for his uncle's demise, and Catherine had accepted with the gracious smile of a lady agreeing to attend a charity function.

Lord Pemberton had died in his sleep three nights later, apparently of a stroke brought on by his notorious temper and fondness for rich food. The physician who examined the body found nothing suspicious, An Dubhán had taught Catherine techniques that left no trace in mortal flesh, methods of killing that mimicked natural death so perfectly that even the most careful investigation would find nothing amiss.

The nephew inherited as expected, paid Catherine's fee without complaint, and recommended her services to certain friends who found themselves in similar difficulties with inconvenient relatives. Within a month, Catherine had orchestrated the deaths of a shipping magnate in Belfast, a banker in Galway, and a judge in Limerick whose verdicts had begun to inconvenience certain criminal enterprises.

Each death was a masterpiece of planning and execution. Catherine would study her targets for weeks, learning their habits and weaknesses, identifying the perfect moment and method for their elimination. She used poisons that An Dubhán whispered in her mind, ancient formulas that modern medicine could not detect, substances that mimicked the symptoms of common ailments so perfectly that no one questioned the deaths that followed.

But it was not just the poisons that made her so effective. Catherine had learned to become what each situation required, a grieving widow seeking comfort, a potential business partner offering lucrative opportunities, a society lady making charitable visits to the sick and elderly. She could be whoever she needed to be, say whatever needed to be said, to gain access to her targets and create the opportunities she required.

The banker in Galway had been particularly satisfying. Patrick O'Sullivan was an Irishman who had grown rich by foreclosing on the farms of his own countrymen, selling their land to English investors while the dispossessed families starved in the ditches. He had been protected by guards and lawyers, surrounded by the wealth that his betrayals had earned him, confident in his security.

Catherine had approached him as the representative of a London syndicate interested in purchasing agricultural properties in the west of Ireland. She had worn her finest dress, spoken in the cultured accent that An Dubhán had taught her, and carried forged credentials that established her as a woman of substantial means and unquestionable respectability. O'Sullivan had welcomed her into his office like a spider welcoming a particularly plump fly into its web.

He had died while reviewing the contracts she had prepared, documents that would have transferred ownership of his assets to phantom companies controlled by Catherine herself. The poison had been worked into the very ink of the papers, An Dubhán's knowledge extended to such sophisticated techniques, and O'Sullivan had absorbed it through his skin as he handled the documents. To all observers, he had simply collapsed from the excitement of concluding such a lucrative transaction.

The authorities had found nothing suspicious. Catherine had played the role of shocked business associate perfectly, even weeping decorously as the body was carried from the office. The contracts, of course, had disappeared in the confusion, and Catherine had departed Galway as mysteriously as she had arrived, leaving behind only the memory of a refined lady who had been tragically present at the scene of an unfortunate natural death.

Each success made the next one easier. Catherine's reputation spread through the networks of the wealthy and desperate, and soon she was receiving offers that would have been unimaginable just months earlier. A consortium of English industrialists wanted her to eliminate a troublesome Irish politician who was advocating for workers' rights. A group of Dublin merchants sought the death of a competitor who was cutting into their profits. Even the Church had use for her services, a bishop privately requested the removal of a priest whose investigations into Church finances had become inconvenient.

The politician died in a carriage accident on the road to Parliament, his horses apparently spooked by a sudden noise in the darkness. The merchant competitor succumbed to what appeared to be food poisoning after dining at his favourite restaurant. The troublesome priest was found dead in his study, apparently having suffered a heart attack while working on his accounts by candlelight.

Catherine moved through these killings like a dancer performing a well-rehearsed ballet, each death flowing seamlessly into the next. She developed a network of contacts, corrupt servants who could provide access to private homes, unscrupulous physicians who would sign death certificates without asking uncomfortable questions, and grave diggers who could ensure that certain bodies were buried quickly and without examination.

An Dubhán grew stronger with each feeding, its presence in Catherine's mind becoming more vivid and substantial. Sometimes she could almost see it, a shadow that moved independently of any earthly form, a darkness that fed on fear and death and the terror of those who realised too late that they had become prey.

"We are creating something beautiful," the creature whispered as Catherine prepared for her next assignment. "A work of art painted in blood and terror, a masterpiece that will be remembered long after these mortal concerns have turned to dust. You are no longer simply killing for money, my dear Catherine. You are reshaping the very fabric of Irish society, removing the obstacles that stand in the way of a better world."

Catherine nodded as she studied the dossier that had been prepared for her latest target. Sir Reginald Ashworth was an English landlord who owned vast estates throughout the Irish countryside. He was known for his cruelty to his tenants, his habit of raising rents beyond what working families could afford, and his practice of evicting entire villages to make way for more profitable sheep pastures. Hundreds of families had been driven from their homes by his greed, left to wander the roads as beggars or die in the workhouses that had become symbols of English indifference to Irish suffering.

But Sir Reginald was also careful, protected by bodyguards and suspicious of strangers. He rarely left his fortified manor house, and when he did venture out, it was always with an armed escort. Previous attempts on his life had failed, leaving behind only the bodies of would-be assassins who had underestimated the precautions that surrounded him.

Catherine smiled as she studied his photograph. Sir Reginald Ashworth would present a challenge worthy of her evolved skills, an opportunity to demonstrate the full extent of what she had become. And the payment, a thousand pounds from a consortium of displaced Irish families who had somehow managed to pool their meagre resources for this one act of vengeance, would be the largest she had ever received.

"How shall we approach this one?" she asked An Dubhán, though she was already beginning to form ideas of her own.

"Patience," the creature replied. "This one requires subtlety and time. But I have been thinking about Sir Reginald's weaknesses, his desires, his vulnerabilities. He is a man who has always taken what he wanted, who has never been denied anything his wealth could purchase. That appetite will be his undoing."

Over the following weeks, Catherine transformed herself once again, this time becoming Lady Victoria Pembroke, a wealthy widow from London with interests in Irish real estate. Her credentials were impeccable, her references unquestionable, her appearance that of a woman who had never known want or hardship. She rented a fashionable house in Dublin and began making the kind of social appearances that would bring her to Sir Reginald's attention.

The plan was audacious in its simplicity. Sir Reginald Ashworth was known for his acquisitive nature, he collected not just land and money, but fine art, rare books, and most especially, beautiful women. He had been married three times, each wife dying under circumstances that had raised whispers but never formal accusations. Lady Victoria Pembroke, with her mysterious past and substantial fortune, would prove irresistible to a man who had never met a treasure he did not wish to possess.

The courtship took months to arrange. Catherine allowed herself to be introduced to Sir Reginald at carefully orchestrated social events, always appearing just out of reach, always suggesting depths of wealth and sophistication that made him eager to know more. She played the role of the unattainable woman perfectly, accepting his invitations with apparent reluctance, allowing his pursuit to build to a fever pitch of desire and determination.

When she finally accepted his proposal of marriage, Sir Reginald Ashworth believed he had won the greatest prize of his acquisitive life. The wedding was to be a grand affair, celebrated at his estate with hundreds of guests from the highest levels of Irish and English society. He had already begun making plans to merge Lady Victoria's supposed fortune with his own, to create an empire of wealth and power that would make him one of the richest men in the British Isles.

Catherine smiled as she listened to his plans, as she toured the estate that would briefly become her home, as she met the servants who would unknowingly assist in their master's destruction. Sir Reginald had no idea that he was not gaining a wife but embracing his own death, that the woman he planned to marry was the instrument of vengeance for all the families he had destroyed, all the lives he had ruined in his relentless pursuit of profit.

The wedding night would be his last night on earth, and Catherine was already planning exactly how he would die. An Dubhán had whispered to her of poisons that worked slowly, that would give a man time to understand what was happening to him, to realise that his wealth and cruelty had finally brought him to this inevitable end.

Sir Reginald Ashworth would die in his marriage bed, alone with his bride and his terror, learning too late that some appetites were more dangerous than others, that some prey turned out to be predators in disguise. And Catherine would emerge from his estate a grieving widow, inheriting his fortune and properties, free to continue her work of reshaping Ireland one death at a time.

The season of blood was far from over. If anything, it was just beginning to reach its full, terrible glory.

The wedding of Sir Reginald Ashworth and Lady Victoria Pembroke was celebrated as the social event of the season. The estate's great hall blazed with candlelight and rang with the laughter of three hundred guests, the cream of Anglo-Irish society gathered to witness what they believed would be the union of two great fortunes. Catherine moved through the celebration like a queen holding court, accepting congratulations with gracious smiles while counting the hours until she could complete her true purpose.

Sir Reginald was in his element, basking in the envy of his peers and the apparent adoration of his beautiful bride. He had consumed enough champagne to loosen his tongue, regaling anyone who would listen with tales of his bride's mysterious fortune and his own cleverness in securing such a prize. Catherine listened to his boasts with the patient attention of a cat watching a mouse, knowing that each word brought him closer to his final breath.

As the evening wore on and the guests gradually departed, Catherine found herself alone with her new husband in the master bedroom of the estate. Sir Reginald had dismissed his servants with unusual haste, eager to claim the ultimate prize of his wedding night. He spoke to Catherine with the casual possession of a man who had never been denied anything he desired, his hands already reaching for her with the confidence of ownership.

"My dear Victoria," he said, his voice thick with wine and anticipation, "you cannot imagine how long I have waited for this moment. You are the crown jewel of my collection, the perfect completion of everything I have built."

Catherine smiled as she poured two glasses of wine from the bottle that had been waiting in their chamber, her movements graceful and unhurried. The wine was a rare vintage from Sir Reginald's own cellars, a fitting medium for the poison that An Dubhán had taught her to distil from the berries of the deadly nightshade. The extract was colourless and nearly tasteless, indistinguishable from the complex flavours of the aged wine.

"To our future together," she said, offering him the poisoned glass while keeping the clean one for herself. "To the joining of our fortunes and the fulfilment of all your desires."

Sir Reginald drank deeply, savouring what he believed would be the wine of victory. Catherine sipped delicately from her own glass, watching as her husband's face began to flush with more than just alcohol and excitement. The poison worked quickly but not mercifully, An Dubhán had chosen a formula that would allow its victim time to understand what was happening, to experience the full terror of approaching death.

"Something is wrong," Sir Reginald said after a few minutes, his hand moving to his throat as his breathing became labored. "I feel... Strange. Hot and cold at the same time."

"Perhaps it's the excitement of the evening," Catherine suggested, moving closer to him with the solicitous concern of a devoted wife. "You have been celebrating rather enthusiastically."

But Sir Reginald was not a stupid man, despite his arrogance and cruelty. As his vision began to blur and his heartbeat became irregular, he looked at Catherine with growing understanding and terror. He tried to speak, to call for help, but his voice emerged as nothing more than a hoarse whisper.

"You," he gasped, his eyes wide with the realisation that he had been outwitted by the woman he had thought to possess. "You're not... You're not Victoria Pembroke."

"No," Catherine agreed, settling herself in a chair beside the bed where her husband lay struggling for each breath. "I am something far more dangerous than a wealthy widow seeking a husband. I am the instrument of justice for every family you have destroyed, every life you have ruined in your greed for land and gold."

Sir Reginald tried to rise from the bed, perhaps hoping to reach the door and summon help, but his muscles would no longer obey his commands. The poison had invaded his nervous system, turning his own body against him with the ruthless efficiency that had characterised all of Catherine"s work.

"The families," he whispered, his voice barely audible. "The families I evicted... They paid you."

"They scraped together their pennies and shillings," Catherine confirmed. "Widows sold their wedding rings, children gave up their only toys, men worked extra jobs for months to contribute to the fund that purchased your death. You are being killed by the collective will of every person you have ever wronged, and there is a beautiful justice in that."

She watched dispassionately as Sir Reginald Ashworth died, his body convulsing with the final spasms of the poison's work. His last expression was one of complete terror and understanding, the look of a man who had finally met a force more ruthless and determined than himself. When his breathing stopped and his eyes grew vacant, Catherine felt the familiar surge of satisfaction that came with a job perfectly executed.

But this time there was something more. As Sir Reginald's spirit departed his body, Catherine could feel An Dubhán feeding with an intensity she had never experienced before. The creature's pleasure flooded through her mind like dark wine, intoxicating and powerful, filling her with a sense of accomplishment that transcended mere professional pride.

"Magnificent," An Dubhán whispered, its voice rich with satisfaction. "You have surpassed even my expectations, my dear Catherine. This was not merely murder, it was artistry, poetry, the perfect fusion of justice and vengeance."

Catherine remained with the body until dawn, playing the role of grieving bride to perfection when the servants finally discovered Sir Reginald's corpse. She wept convincingly at the inquest, spoke movingly of her brief happiness and sudden loss, and accepted the condolences of the community with the dignity expected of a woman of her apparent station.

The authorities found nothing suspicious about Sir Reginald's death. The physician attributed it to heart failure brought on by the excitement of his wedding night and his well-known tendency toward excess. Catherine inherited everything, the estate, the fortune, the properties scattered across Ireland that represented decades of exploitation and cruelty.

But she had no intention of keeping her inheritance. Within a month of Sir Reginald's funeral, Catherine had transferred ownership of all his properties to a trust that would distribute the land to the families who had been evicted from it. The money she kept, adding it to the growing fortune that funded her increasingly ambitious operations.

News of Sir Reginald's death and the mysterious redistribution of his wealth spread through Ireland like wildfire. The dispossessed families who suddenly found themselves with legal title to their ancestral lands spoke of it as a miracle, a sign that justice could still prevail in a world that seemed designed to favour the cruel and the greedy. But in the drawing rooms and private clubs where the wealthy and powerful gathered, there were darker whispers about the widow who had appeared from nowhere and vanished just as mysteriously, leaving behind only questions and a growing sense of unease.

Catherine had become more than just a killer for hire. She was becoming something like a force of nature, a correction to the imbalances that had made Irish society a playground for English exploitation. The wealthy began to look over their shoulders, to question the loyalty of their servants, to wonder if they too might become targets of whatever power had struck down one of their most protected members.

The fear was intoxicating. Catherine could taste it in the air at social gatherings, could see it in the eyes of men who had always believed their money could buy them safety from any consequence. They invited her to their parties, still believing her to be Lady Victoria Pembroke, the mysterious widow of the late Sir Reginald, but they watched her with the nervous attention of prey animals sensing a predator nearby.

An Dubhán revelled in their terror. The creature's appetite had grown enormous, fed by the fear that preceded each killing and the satisfaction that followed. It began to demand more frequent feedings, more elaborate schemes, targets that would create greater ripples of panic through the networks of the privileged and corrupt.

"There is a gathering next month," the creature whispered as Catherine counted the latest payment from grateful clients. "A secret meeting of the most powerful landlords in Ireland, men who coordinate their policies of exploitation and oppression. They meet to divide the country among themselves, to plan new methods of extracting wealth from the people they have conquered."

Catherine felt her pulse quicken with anticipation. "How many will be there?"

"Twelve of the wealthiest and most influential men in Ireland," An Dubhán replied, its voice rich with dark promise. “All gathered in one place, all vulnerable to someone with your particular talents. Imagine the terror when they begin dying one by one, when their secret conclave becomes a charnel house.”

The plan that emerged from their collaboration was ambitious beyond anything Catherine had attempted before. Rather than killing her targets individually over months or years, she would eliminate an entire conspiracy in a single night, striking at the very heart of the system that had oppressed Ireland for centuries.

The gathering was to take place at Blackwater Castle, an ancient fortress on the coast of County Cork that had been converted into a private retreat for the Anglo-Irish aristocracy. The twelve landlords would spend three days in isolation, planning their strategies for the coming year without fear of interference or observation. They would bring minimal staff, rely on the castle’s remote location for security, and never suspect that their greatest enemy was already among them.

Catherine spent weeks preparing for the operation. She studied the castle’s layout, identified the servants who could be bribed or intimidated into cooperation, and developed a dozen different methods for killing that would appear to be accidents or natural deaths. Most importantly, she cultivated a new identity, Lady Margaret Thornfield, a recently widowed plantation owner from the West Indies with interests in Irish agricultural investments.

The transformation was her most complete yet. Lady Margaret was older than Catherine's previous personas, distinguished by silver-streaked hair and the bearing of someone accustomed to command. Her accent carried hints of colonial sophistication, her knowledge of sugar cultivation and slave management was encyclopedic, and her credentials were impeccable enough to gain her entry to the most exclusive circles of Anglo-Irish society.

When Lady Margaret Thornfield arrived at Blackwater Castle for the secret conclave, she was welcomed as a valuable addition to their conspiracy. The twelve landlords saw in her the promise of new investment opportunities, new methods of exploitation that had been perfected in the sugar islands and could be adapted to Irish conditions. They had no idea that they were welcoming death itself into their sanctuary, that the woman they hoped to learn from was planning to make their gathering a monument to the justice they had so long denied.

The first death came on the second night of the conclave. Lord Pembroke, a different Pembroke than the one whose identity Catherine had briefly assumed, was found dead in his bed, apparently having choked on his own vomit after drinking too heavily at dinner. It was an undignified end for a man who prided himself on his refinement, but the others assumed it was merely an unfortunate accident.

The second death followed within hours. Sir William Crawford, a notorious rack-renter from County Antrim, was discovered at the bottom of the castle's main staircase with his neck broken. The stone steps were worn smooth by centuries of use, and it seemed plausible that an elderly man might lose his footing in the darkness and fall to his death.

But when the third man died, Lord Ashton, found floating face-down in the castle's ornamental pond, the survivors began to understand that they were under attack by something far more dangerous than bad luck or coincidence. They gathered in the castle's great hall like sheep huddling together for protection, their voices rising in panic as they debated whether to flee or send for help.

Catherine watched their terror with the detached interest of a natural philosopher observing an interesting experiment. She had poisoned Lord Pembroke's brandy with a delayed-action toxin that would not take effect until hours after consumption. She had loosened the stone balustrade on the staircase and left oil on the steps where Sir William was certain to slip. Lord Ashton's death had been the most direct, a simple matter of striking him unconscious and holding his head underwater until his struggles ceased.

An Dubhán was feeding voraciously on the fear that filled the castle like fog. The creature's presence in Catherine's mind had become almost overwhelming, its hunger satisfied beyond anything it had experienced in centuries. Each death fed it, each moment of terror sustained it, each desperate prayer for salvation from the surviving conspirators only strengthened its connection to the mortal world.

"More," the creature whispered, its voice thick with satisfaction. "We must have more. They are beginning to understand the magnitude of their situation, and their fear is becoming exquisite."

Catherine smiled as she prepared for the next phase of her plan. Nine men remained alive in the castle, nine powerful figures who had spent their lives inflicting suffering on others and were now discovering what it felt like to be helpless prey. Before the sun rose again, Blackwater Castle would become a tomb for the entire conspiracy, a monument to the price of oppression that would send shockwaves throughout the Anglo-Irish establishment.

The season of blood was reaching its crescendo, and Catherine Blackthorne had become death incarnate, a force of nature disguised as a lady of quality. The weight of stones that had shaped her childhood had been transformed into something far more deadly, the weight of justice, falling like an avalanche on those who had earned their destruction through a lifetime of cruelty and greed.

Chapter Six
My Brother's Ghost

Catherine Blackthorne stood among the corpses in Blackwater Castle's great hall, surveying her night's work with the satisfaction of an artist contemplating a completed masterpiece. Nine more bodies lay scattered throughout the ancient fortress, some poisoned, some apparently victims of accidents, all dead by her hand. The conspiracy that had gathered to divide Ireland among themselves had been permanently dissolved, their plans buried with them in the cold stone chambers where they had thought themselves safe from consequence.

An Dubhán's presence in her mind was stronger than it had ever been, gorged on the fear and death that had saturated the castle through the long night. The creature's satisfaction radiated through Catherine's consciousness like warm honey, sweet with the taste of perfect revenge and flawless execution.

But as dawn began to creep through the tall windows, casting pale light across the scene of slaughter, something changed. The air in the great hall grew suddenly cold, colder than the Irish winter had any right to be. Frost began to form on the stone walls, and Catherine's breath misted in the suddenly frigid atmosphere.

"What," she began, but the words died in her throat as a familiar figure materialised at the far end of the hall.

Padraig Costello stood there as he had in life, but translucent now, wreathed in mist that seemed to rise from the very stones beneath his feet. His face bore the same expression Catherine remembered from their final moments together in the grove, surprise, pain, and a terrible understanding. But there was something else in his ghostly features now, something that made her blood run cold despite all the death she had dealt and witnessed.

"Hello, sister," he said, his voice carrying across the hall like wind through empty graves. "It's been a long time."

Catherine felt An Dubhán recoil within her mind, the creature's presence suddenly diminished, as if it were trying to hide from something it found threatening or distasteful. For the first time since their partnership began, Catherine sensed fear in the ancient thing that had made her into an instrument of death.

"You're not real," Catherine said, though even as she spoke the words, she knew they were a lie. "I killed you twenty years ago. You're dead and gone."

"Dead, yes," Padraig agreed, his form becoming more solid as he spoke. "But not gone. Never gone. Did you think that striking a bargain with that shadow would free you from what you did? Did you imagine that becoming something other than Mary Costello would wash the blood from your hands?"

Other figures began to materialise around the great hall, Cormac with his skull caved in from the stone that had sent him over the bridge, Brigid with her lips blue from the poisoned water, their father Seamus with his face grey from drink and despair. All the ghosts that had vanished when Catherine first accepted An Dubhán's offer now stood among the fresh corpses, their eyes fixed on the woman who had once been their sister and daughter.

"We've been waiting," Cormac said, his voice a wet whisper that seemed to come from the bottom of a deep well. "Waiting for you to remember what you truly are beneath all these fine clothes and false names."

"You cannot escape your nature, Mary," Brigid added, her form flickering like candlelight in a draft. "You can call yourself Catherine or Victoria or Margaret, but you will always be the girl who murdered her family and fed their souls to darkness."Catherine felt something she had not experienced in years, genuine fear. These were not the sad, resigned spirits that had once haunted her cottage. These ghosts burned with an anger that seemed to make the very air around them writhe and twist. They had grown stronger during their absence, fed by some power that rivalled or perhaps exceeded An Dubhán's ancient hunger.

"What do you want?" Catherine asked, her voice barely steady.

"Justice," Seamus Costello replied, his ghostly form towering over his daughter with the same authority he had wielded in life. "For twenty years, you have escaped the consequences of your crimes against your own blood. But debts must be paid, Mary. The ledger must be balanced."

An Dubhán stirred uneasily in Catherine's mind, its whisper now uncertain where once it had been confident. "This is unexpected," the creature admitted. "These spirits should not have the power to manifest so strongly, should not be able to penetrate the protections I have woven around you."

"Your protections?" Padraig laughed, the sound like glass breaking in a church. "You think your power can shield her from what she owes us? You are old, shadow-thing, but we are older. We are the first debts she created, the original sins that made all the rest possible. And we have been growing stronger while she grew fat on other people's deaths."

Catherine looked around the great hall, seeing it now through different eyes. The corpses of the landlords suddenly seemed less like victories and more like evidence,proof of what she had become, of how far she had travelled from the desperate girl who had killed to protect herself. Each death had been a step further into darkness, each success a deeper betrayal of whatever humanity she might once have possessed.

"I became what I needed to become," Catherine said, but her voice lacked the conviction it had once carried. "I survived. I turned my suffering into strength."

"You turned your pain into poison," Brigid corrected her. "You let that creature twist you into something that feeds on death like a carrion bird. Look at yourself, Mary. Look at what you've become."

For the first time in years, Catherine did look, truly look, at what she had made of herself. She saw the elegant clothes that disguised a killer, the refined manners that masked a predator, the beautiful face that had lured dozens of victims to their deaths. She had become magnificent and terrible, exactly as An Dubhán had promised. But she had also become something that her family, murdered though they were, could barely recognise as human.

"The shadow offered you power," Seamus said, his ghostly eyes boring into his daughter's soul. "But it never told you the price, did it? Every life you take in its service makes you less yourself and more its creature. Soon there will be nothing left of Mary Costello except the shell that carries out its will."

An Dubhán's presence flared with sudden anger. "Lies!" the creature snarled in Catherine's mind. "They seek to poison you against our partnership, to make you doubt the glory we have achieved together. You are more than you have ever been, more powerful, more feared, more"

"More empty," Padraig interrupted, apparently able to hear the creature's words. "More hollow with each passing day. Tell me, sister, when did you last feel genuine emotion? When did you last experience anything but the cold satisfaction of a successful kill? When did you last remember what it felt like to be human?"

Catherine opened her mouth to answer, then closed it again as she realised she had no response. When had she last felt real joy, real sorrow, real love or hate or fear that belonged to her rather than to the ancient thing that shared her thoughts? The emotions she had experienced in recent years had all been calculated, performed, and designed to serve her purposes rather than express her true feelings.

"You see?" Cormac said gently. "The shadow has been eating you from the inside, consuming everything that made you Mary Costello and replacing it with its own hunger. Soon you will be nothing but a hollow vessel for its appetite, and then even death will not free you from what you have become."

"But there is another way," Brigid added, stepping closer to her sister with something that might have been compassion in her ghostly features. "A chance to reclaim what you have lost, to remember who you were before the shadow claimed you."

Catherine felt An Dubhán writhing in her mind like a serpent caught in a trap. The creature's voice, when it came, was desperate and commanding at once. "Do not listen to them! They offer only weakness and suffering, the same pain that drove you to seek my partnership in the first place. With me, you are powerful beyond measure. Without me, you are nothing but a peasant girl destined for poverty and abuse."

"Perhaps," Seamus said, apparently still able to hear the creature's words. "But she would be herself again. She would be human again, with all the pain and weakness that entails. The question is whether she has the courage to choose humanity over power, whether any part of Mary Costello still exists beneath the mask of Catherine Blackthorne."

Catherine looked around the great hall one more time, seeing the corpses of the landlords, the ghostly forms of her family, the pale light of dawn filtering through windows that had witnessed centuries of violence and conspiracy. She felt the weight of An Dubhán's presence in her mind, the creature's power flowing through her like dark wine. She had never been stronger, never been more capable of imposing her will upon the world.

But she had also never been more alone. The ghosts of her victims no longer visited her, An Dubhán had dismissed them as unnecessary distractions. The living feared her too much to offer genuine companionship. Even her triumphs felt hollow, mechanical, like the movements of a clockwork figure wound tight and set to its predetermined course.

"What are you offering me?" Catherine asked her family's ghosts, though she suspected she already knew the answer.

"A choice," Padraig said simply. "Break free from the shadow's influence, accept the consequences of what you have done, and find whatever redemption might still be possible for someone who has travelled as far into darkness as you have. It will not be easy, and it may not be pleasant. But it will be real in a way that nothing has been real for you in years."

"And if I refuse?"

"Then you continue as you are," Brigid replied. "Growing ever more hollow, ever more lost, until the day comes when the shadow no longer needs even the pretence of partnership. You will become its creature entirely, and Mary Costello will be as dead as if you had never drawn breath."

An Dubhán's voice rose to a shriek in Catherine's mind. ""She lies! They all lie! You are meant for greatness, for power that transcends mortal understanding! Do not throw away everything we have built together for the sake of sentiment and guilt!"

But even as the creature raged, Catherine could feel its hold on her weakening. The presence of her family's ghosts seemed to be creating cracks in the prison of power that An Dubhán had built around her soul. For the first time in years, she could remember what it had felt like to be simply Mary Costello, frightened, angry, desperate, but undeniably human.

The choice hung before her like a sword balanced on its point. Power or humanity. The creature's strength or her own soul. The magnificent emptiness of Catherine Blackthorne or the painful reality of Mary Costello.

In the growing light of dawn, surrounded by the dead and the ghostly, Catherine closed her eyes and made her decision.

"Forgive me," she whispered, though she was not entirely sure to whom she was speaking, her family's ghosts, her victims, or the lost girl she had once been. "Forgive me, and help me find my way back to whatever I was before the shadow claimed me."

An Dubhán's scream of rage and betrayal echoed through the great hall like the sound of a world ending. But as Catherine felt the creature's power beginning to tear itself free from her mind, she also felt something else, a warmth she had not experienced in decades, the first stirring of what might, with time and effort and perhaps a kind of grace she did not deserve, eventually become hope.

Chapter Seven
The Unmaking

The pain of separation was beyond anything Mary had ever imagined. As An Dubhán's power tore itself free from her mind, she felt as though her very soul was being flayed, layer by layer, until nothing remained but raw, bleeding consciousness. The creature's departure was not gentle, it ripped away pieces of her memory, her knowledge, her carefully constructed identity, leaving behind wounds that burned like acid in her thoughts.

She collapsed to the stone floor of Blackwater Castle's great hall, her elegant dress torn and stained with blood from the corpses that surrounded her. The refined posture that had marked Catherine Blackthorne crumbled, replaced by the hunched shoulders and defensive crouch of Mary Costello, the abused girl who had learned to make herself small in the face of violence.

An Dubhán's final scream echoed through the castle like the death cry of some ancient god, filled with rage and betrayal and a hunger that would never again be satisfied through her actions. The sound seemed to go on forever, reverberating through dimensions that human ears were never meant to perceive, until it finally faded into the kind of silence that follows the end of the world.

"It is done," Seamus Costello's ghost said, his voice gentler now than it had been in life or death. "The shadow is banished, its hold on you broken. But the work is far from over, daughter. Now comes the harder task, learning to live with what you have done while that thing wore your face."

Mary looked up at her father's spirit with eyes that streamed tears she had not shed in twenty years. The elegant composure of Catherine Blackthorne was gone, stripped away along with An Dubhán's power, leaving behind only the raw humanity that had been buried beneath layers of sophisticated cruelty.

"I remember," she whispered, her voice cracking with the weight of returning emotion. "I remember everything. Every death, every moment of terror, every life I snuffed out like a candle flame. God help me, I remember it all."

"Good," Brigid said, kneeling beside her sister with a tenderness that seemed impossible from someone Mary had murdered decades ago. "Memory is the beginning of conscience, and conscience is the beginning of redemption, if redemption is even possible for someone who has done what you have done."

The knowledge that An Dubhán had poured into Mary's mind was fading like mist before the morning sun. The sophisticated poisons, the methods of killing that left no trace, the social graces that had allowed Catherine Blackthorne to move through high society—all of it was draining away, leaving Mary with nothing but her native cunning and the terrible weight of her crimes.

But something else was returning to fill the void left by the creature's departure. Emotions she had not felt in years began to stir in her chest, guilt, shame, horror at what she had become, but also something that might, with time, grow into genuine remorse. For the first time since she had struck Padraig with that stone in the grove, Mary Costello felt truly, completely human.

"What happens now?" she asked, struggling to her feet on legs that shook with more than just physical weakness. "The authorities will come looking for the men who died here. They'll want answers, investigations, justice."

"Then give them justice," Padraig said, his ghostly form beginning to fade as dawn fully broke through the castle's windows. "Give them the truth, sister. Tell them what Catherine Blackthorne really was, what Mary Costello became. Accept the consequences of your choices."

"They'll hang me," Mary said, but there was no fear in her voice now, only a strange kind of relief. "Or transport me to the colonies if I'm fortunate. Either way, my life as I've known it is over."

"Your life as Catherine Blackthorne is over," Cormac corrected her. "But Mary Costello's story may yet have chapters unwritten. The choice of how to fill them is yours, but it must be your choice this time, not the shadow's, not circumstances', not desperation's. Yours alone."

The ghosts of her family were becoming more translucent with each passing moment, their forms dissolving like salt in water. But before they faded entirely, Seamus stepped forward and placed what felt like a real hand on his daughter's shoulder.

"We forgive you," he said simply. "For what that means, for what it's worth after all these years, we forgive you, Mary. The question now is whether you can forgive yourself, and whether the world you've helped to darken can ever find light again."

And then they were gone, leaving Mary alone among the corpses with nothing but the growing daylight and the weight of decisions that could no longer be delayed or delegated to ancient powers with their own agendas.

She walked slowly through Blackwater Castle, seeing it now through eyes unclouded by An Dubhán's influence. The bodies of the landlords lay where she had left them, but they no longer looked like trophies or artistic statements. They looked like what they were, dead human beings, cut down in the prime of their lives by someone who had convinced herself that murder could serve justice.

Some of them had been cruel, yes. Greedy and exploitative, certainly. But they had also been fathers and husbands, sons and brothers, men with their own stories and struggles and perhaps even their own chances for redemption, chances she had stolen from them in service to a creature that fed on death and terror.

Mary found paper and ink in the castle's library and sat down to write the most difficult letter of her life. It was addressed to the magistrates of Cork, a full confession of everything Catherine Blackthorne had done, every life she had taken, every crime she had committed in service to An Dubhán's hunger. She wrote until her hand cramped and her eyes burned, setting down in careful detail the methods she had used, the victims she had claimed, the network of corruption and conspiracy she had exploited to carry out her work.

When it was finished, the confession ran to nearly thirty pages of closely written text. It was a complete indictment of everything she had become, a roadmap to every secret she had kept, every false identity she had assumed, every death she had arranged. It would destroy whatever reputation Catherine Blackthorne had built and ensure that Mary Costello faced the full consequences of her actions.

But as she sealed the letter and prepared to send it on its way to Cork, Mary felt something she had not experienced in decades, a sense of completion, of honesty, of finally telling the truth after years of living in elaborate lies. The weight of secrets that had pressed down on her for so long was lifting, replaced by a different kind of weight, the weight of responsibility, of accountability, of facing the world as she truly was rather than as she had pretended to be.

The castle's surviving servants had fled during the night, terrified by the sounds of death and the supernatural cold that had filled the building during her confrontation with the ghosts. Mary was alone with the dead, which seemed fitting somehow. She had spent so much of her life surrounded by corpses of her own making that solitude among them felt almost natural.

She spent her final hours of freedom walking through the Irish countryside around Blackwater Castle, seeing it as if for the first time. The hills rolled away toward the distant sea, green and brown and beautiful in the morning light. Farmers worked their fields, children played by stone walls, and women hung laundry to dry in the salt-scented breeze. It was a world she had moved through but never truly inhabited, focused as she had been on death and revenge and the satisfaction of An Dubhán's endless hunger.

But now, with the creature's influence gone and her family's forgiveness burning in her heart like a coal, Mary could see the beauty and possibility that surrounded her. Not that it mattered, her part in this world was ending, and ending by her own choice. But there was comfort in knowing that life would continue after her, that the sun would still rise and set, that people would still love and hope and dream despite everything she had done to darken their world.

When the constables came for her the next morning, summoned by her confession and the discovery of the bodies in Blackwater Castle, Mary was waiting for them in the castle's great hall. She had cleaned the blood from the floor as best she could and arranged the corpses with what dignity remained to them. She was dressed in a simple black dress she had found in the servants' quarters, her hair pinned back plainly, her face free of the cosmetics that had helped create Catherine Blackthorne's mask of beauty.

"Are you Mary Costello?" the chief constable asked, his hand resting on the pistol at his belt.

"I am," Mary replied simply. "I've been waiting for you."

They bound her hands with iron shackles that felt surprisingly light after the invisible chains that An Dubhán had wrapped around her soul for so many years. As they led her from Blackwater Castle toward the cart that would carry her to Cork for trial, Mary looked back once at the ancient fortress where her old life had finally ended.

The morning sun was shining through the windows of the great hall, illuminating the spaces where her family's ghosts had appeared to offer her one last chance at redemption. The light seemed warmer than it had any right to be, full of possibilities that Mary would never live to see but that might, perhaps, exist because of the choice she had made to embrace her humanity over her power.

For the first time in twenty years, Mary Costello was truly free. Free from An Dubhán's whispers, free from the need to pretend she was someone else, free from the weight of secrets that had bent her soul nearly to breaking. The freedom would be brief, she would hang for her crimes, and hang deservedly, but it was real in a way that nothing had been real for her in decades.

As the cart rolled toward Cork and whatever justice awaited her there, Mary closed her eyes and felt the Irish sun warm on her face. She was going to die, probably soon, probably badly. But she was going to die as herself, and after everything that had happened, that seemed like the most precious gift she could have asked for.

The unmaking was complete. What remained to be seen was whether anything worth preserving could rise from the ruins of what she had become.

Chapter Eight
The Reckoning

The trial of Mary Costello became the sensation of Ireland. In the autumn of 1847, while the country still reeled from the devastation of the potato famine, the courtroom in Cork was packed daily with spectators hungry for details of the crimes that had terrorised the Anglo-Irish establishment. Newspapers from Dublin to London sent their best reporters to cover what they called "The Black Widow Murders," though none of them truly understood the scope of what had been revealed in Mary's confession.

Mary sat in the dock wearing the same simple black dress she had been arrested in, her hands folded calmly in her lap, her face bearing an expression of serene resignation that unnerved everyone who looked upon her. Gone was any trace of Catherine Blackthorne's sophisticated beauty or Lady Victoria Pembroke's aristocratic bearing. This was Mary Costello as she truly was, a peasant woman of middle years, worn by hard living and harder choices, facing the consequences of two decades of methodical murder.

The prosecutor, Sir Edmund Harwick, was a theatrical man who understood that this case would make or break his career. He paced before the jury like a stalking cat, his voice rising and falling as he painted Mary as a monster disguised in human form, a creature of such calculated evil that her very existence challenged the natural order of civilised society.

“Gentlemen of the jury,” he declared on the opening day of testimony, “you are asked to judge not merely a murderess, but something far more dangerous, a woman who has made an art of death, who has turned killing into a profession as refined as any practised by the most skilled craftsman. The defendant has confessed to no fewer than thirty-seven murders, each one planned with meticulous care, each one executed with a precision that speaks to a mind utterly devoid of human conscience.”

Mary listened to the recitation of her crimes with the detachment of someone hearing about the actions of a stranger. In many ways, that was exactly what she was doing. The woman who had poisoned Magistrate Blackwood, who had orchestrated the slaughter at Blackwater Castle, who had moved through Irish society like death in an evening gown, that woman felt like someone she had once known but could barely remember.

The evidence against her was overwhelming. Her detailed confession provided a roadmap to every murder, every false identity, every method she had employed. Witnesses came forward to testify about Catherine Blackthorne’s presence at social gatherings where victims had later died under mysterious circumstances. Servants identified her as Lady Victoria Pembroke, the grieving widow who had inherited Sir Reginald Ashworth’s estate only to give it all away to his former tenants.

But it was not the evidence that fascinated the crowds who packed the courtroom each day. It was Mary herself, her calm acceptance of her fate, her refusal to offer any defence or explanation beyond the simple truth she had already revealed. When the prosecutor demanded to know why she had turned to murder, why she had embraced such systematic evil, Mary's answer was as direct as it was unsatisfying.

"I was broken," she said simply, her voice carrying clearly through the hushed courtroom. "Broken by my childhood, broken by poverty and abuse and the weight of simply surviving in a world that had no place for someone like me. Something found me in that brokenness, something old and hungry and patient, and it offered me power in exchange for becoming its instrument. I accepted that bargain, and thirty-seven people died because of my choice.""But surely," Sir Edmund pressed, "you understood that what you were doing was wrong? You knew these people were innocent of any crimes against you personally?"

Mary considered the question with the same careful attention she had once given to planning murders. "Some were innocent," she agreed. "Others were not. Magistrate Blackwood had sentenced innocent men to death for crimes they did not commit. Sir Reginald Ashworth had driven hundreds of families from their homes to starve in ditches. The landlords at Blackwater Castle had conspired to extract every last penny from people who were already dying of hunger."

A murmur ran through the courtroom at this. Many of the spectators were Irish, and the names Mary mentioned were well-known to them, symbols of the oppression and exploitation that had made the famine worse than it needed to be.

"But that does not justify murder," Sir Edmund countered. "No matter how guilty these men may have been of cruelty or greed, they deserved to face justice through proper legal channels, not to be struck down by a self-appointed executioner."

"You're right," Mary said, and the simple admission seemed to take some of the wind out of the prosecutor's sails. "They deserved better than they got from me. They deserved the chance to change, to make amends, to face their victims and their God with whatever accountability they could muster. I stole that chance from them, and I stole it not for justice but because I had become something that fed on death and terror. That is my crime, and I accept full responsibility for it."

The trial continued for three weeks, but its outcome was never in doubt. Mary's confession was complete and detailed, her guilt undeniable, her refusal to mount any meaningful defence tantamount to a plea for the ultimate punishment. The jury deliberated for less than an hour before returning with its verdict.

"Guilty on all counts," the foreman announced, his voice barely steady. "And we recommend that the defendant be sentenced to death by hanging."

Judge Morrison, a severe man with steel-gray hair and eyes like winter frost, looked down at Mary from his bench with an expression that might have been pity if pity had any place in a courtroom dealing with such systematic evil.

"Mary Costello," he said formally, "you have been found guilty of thirty-seven counts of murder in the first degree. You have confessed to crimes that shock the conscience and challenge the very foundations of civilised society. You have shown no remorse for your actions and no indication that you would refrain from similar acts if given the opportunity."

Mary stood to receive her sentence with the same calm composure she had maintained throughout the trial. She felt no fear of death, after everything she had done, it seemed like the most natural conclusion to her story. What surprised her was the sense of peace that had settled over her in recent weeks, a tranquillity born of finally telling the truth after so many years of elaborate deception.

"It is the judgment of this court," Judge Morrison continued, "that you be taken from here to Kilmainham Gaol, there to await execution by hanging. May God have mercy on your soul, though I fear you have placed yourself beyond the reach of any earthly mercy."

Mary inclined her head slightly, accepting the sentence as she had accepted everything else, with the dignity of someone who had finally learned to take responsibility for her choices.

But as the guards moved forward to escort her from the courtroom, a commotion erupted in the gallery. An elderly woman in a worn but clean dress stood up, her voice carrying clearly through the chamber despite her obvious frailty.

"Wait," she called out, her Irish accent thick with emotion. "Please, Your Honour, I must speak."

Judge Morrison frowned at the interruption, but something in the woman's manner gave him pause. "Who

are you, madam, and what business do you have with this court?"

"My name is Kathleen Murphy," the woman replied, her hands shaking as she gripped the gallery rail. "My husband was Seamus Murphy, one of Sir Reginald Ashworth's tenants. We were evicted from our farm three years ago, left to starve by the roadside with our six children."

A hush fell over the courtroom as the woman continued speaking, her voice growing stronger with each word.

"Sir Reginald's agents came in the middle of winter, threw us out of the home my family had worked for three generations. My youngest, little Michael, died of the cold before we could find shelter. My husband, he tried to find work, tried to keep us fed, but there was nothing for an Irish farmer whose land had been stolen. He died of despair, Your Honour. Just lay down one night and never woke up."

Tears were streaming down her face now, but her voice remained steady.

"When we heard that Sir Reginald was dead, when we learned that our farm had been given back to us by his mysterious widow, we thought it was a miracle. My surviving children, they have a home again because of what this woman did. I don't know if that makes it right, but I thought the court should know, some of the people she killed, they left behind more than grieving families. They left behind victims who were finally free."

Judge Morrison stared at the woman for a long moment, his stern expression softening slightly. Around

the courtroom, other voices began to rise, tenants who had been evicted, workers who had been cheated of wages, families who had lost loved ones to the greed and cruelty of Mary's victims.

"Silence!" the judge called, rapping his gavel sharply against the bench. "This court will not be turned into a forum for vigilante justice. Whatever crimes these men may have committed, they did not deserve to be murdered in their beds."

But the damage was done. The moral clarity that had seemed so absolute during the trial was now muddied by the testimony of those who had suffered under the system that Mary's victims had represented. The crowd that filed out of the courtroom was subdued, thoughtful, wrestling with questions that had no easy answers.

Mary was led away to Kilmainham Gaol in chains, but she carried with her the memory of Kathleen Murphy's words, the knowledge that at least some small good had come from the evil she had done. It was not redemption, she was too clear-eyed about her crimes to believe that was possible, but it was something. A reminder that even the darkest actions could cast shadows that fell in unexpected directions, that the world was more complex than the simple categories of good and evil that she had tried to impose upon it.

As the prison gates closed behind her, Mary Costello began the final chapter of her story. She had three weeks to live before the executioner's rope would end her life, three weeks to come to terms with everything she had done and everything she had failed to do.

In the darkness of her cell, surrounded by stone walls that had held generations of Irish rebels and criminals, Mary closed her eyes and tried to remember what it had felt like to be human before An Dubhán had found her. The memories were faint but growing stronger, like stars emerging as night deepened.

She had chosen truth over power, humanity over the creature's promises, justice over the easy path of continued deception. Now all that remained was to see if she could find peace in the time that remained to her, and perhaps, though she barely dared hope for it, some small measure of forgiveness from the God she had spent so many years defying.

The walls of Kilmainham Gaol wept constantly, moisture from the Dublin air condensing on ancient stones that had absorbed decades of human misery. Mary's cell was barely eight feet square, furnished with nothing but a straw mattress, a wooden bucket, and a small barred window that admitted a rectangle of grey light during the day. It was here, in this tomb for the living, that she would spend her remaining time on earth.

The other prisoners treated her with a mixture of fear and fascination. Word of her crimes had spread through the gaol like wildfire, growing more lurid with each telling. Some whispered that she had made a pact with the devil himself, that she could kill with a glance or a touch. Others claimed she was a kind of avenging angel, striking down the oppressors of Ireland with divine fury. The truth, as always, was more complex and less satisfying than the legends that grew around it.

Father O'Malley arrived on Mary's third day in the gaol. He was a young priest, barely thirty, with the kind of earnest idealism that had not yet been worn away by years of ministering to the desperate and the damned. He carried himself with the confidence of someone who believed that no soul was beyond redemption, that even the most hardened criminal could find their way back to grace through sincere repentance.

"Mrs. Costello," he said, settling himself on the single wooden stool that served as the cell's only furniture. "I've come to offer you spiritual counsel in your final days. I understand you were raised in the Catholic faith?"

Mary looked at him from her place on the straw mattress, noting the way he held himself slightly apart from her, as if her proximity might contaminate him with whatever evil he believed she carried.

"I was," she replied simply. "Though I fear I've strayed rather far from the teachings of my childhood, Father."

"No one strays so far that they cannot find their way home," Father O'Malley said with the conviction of youth and inexperience. "Christ died for all sinners, even those who have committed the gravest crimes. Repentance and absolution are available to anyone with a truly contrite heart."

Mary almost smiled at his certainty. Once, she might have found comfort in such simple faith, in the belief that forgiveness was just a prayer away. But she had seen too much, done too much, to believe that salvation could be purchased so easily.

"Tell me, Father," she said, "do you believe that some sins are unforgivable? That there are crimes so terrible that they place the perpetrator beyond God's mercy?"

The young priest shifted uncomfortably on his stool. This was not the conversation he had expected to have with a condemned murderess. He had come prepared to offer comfort to a broken woman, not to engage in theological debates with someone who spoke with the calm certainty of long experience.

"The Church teaches that God's mercy is infinite," he said carefully. "But it also teaches that repentance must be genuine, that the sinner must truly understand the gravity of their crimes and feel authentic remorse for them."

"And if they do? If they understand completely what they've done and accept full responsibility for it, but cannot brng themselves to feel the kind of crushing guilt that everyone expects?" Mary's voice was gentle, curious, as if she were discussing an abstract philosophical problem rather than her own damnation.

Father O'Malley stared at her for a long moment, his young face creased with concentration as he tried to understand what she was asking him.

"Do you feel no remorse for what you've done?" he asked finally.

Mary considered the question with the same careful attention she had once given to planning murders. "I feel sorrow," she said eventually. "Sorrow for the pain I've caused to innocent family members, for the opportunities I've stolen from my victims, for the fear I've spread through communities that had troubles enough without adding me to them. But remorse... Crushing, soul-destroying guilt... No, Father. I can't honestly say I feel that."

"But why?" The question burst from him with genuine anguish. "Thirty-seven people died by your hand. How can you sit here so calmly, speaking of sorrow as if you were discussing the weather?"

Mary was quiet for so long that Father O'Malley began to wonder if she had fallen asleep. When she finally spoke, her voice was so soft he had to lean forward to hear her.

"Because I spent twenty years learning not to feel, Father. Learning to bury my emotions so deeply that they couldn't interfere with what I believed was necessary work. An Dubhán, the thing that guided me, it fed on death and terror, but it also fed on the part of me that might have hesitated, that might have chosen mercy over efficiency. By the time I broke free from its influence, the capacity for the kind of guilt you expect from me had been... Cauterized. Burned away."

She looked up at him then, and Father O'Malley saw something in her eyes that chilled him more than any expression of defiant evil could have. He saw emptiness, not the emptiness of someone who had never felt emotion, but the hollowed-out void left behind when natural human feeling had been systematically destroyed.

"I know what I did was wrong," Mary continued. "I know it intellectually, morally, spiritually. I accept that I deserve to die for it, and I'm prepared to face whatever judgment awaits me beyond death. But I cannot manufacture feelings I no longer possess, Father, not even to ease your mind or my own."

The priest left that day without offering absolution, though he promised to return. Mary watched him go with something approaching pity. He would struggle with her case, would pray and consult his superiors and lose sleep over the question of whether salvation was possible for someone who understood their crimes but could not properly repent them.

Other visitors came in the days that followed. Journalists seeking interviews for their sensational stories, though Mary refused to speak with them. Curiosity seekers hoping for a glimpse of the infamous Black Widow were turned away by the guards. Even a few members of the Anglo-Irish establishment, men who wanted to look into the face of the woman who had terrorized their class for so long.

But the visitor who surprised her most was Kathleen Murphy, the elderly woman who had spoken at her trial. She arrived on a grey Thursday morning, carrying a basket covered with a checkered cloth and wearing the same worn but clean dress she had worn to court.

"I brought you some food," she said simply, settling herself on the stool with the ease of someone accustomed to hard chairs and uncomfortable circumstances. "Prison fare is hardly fit for pigs, and I thought you might appreciate something made with care."

Mary stared at her in confusion. "Why would you do that? You know what I am, what I've done."

"I know you killed Sir Reginald Ashworth," Kathleen replied, unpacking bread, cheese and hard-boiled eggs from her basket. “And I know that because you did, my children have their farm back and food on their table. I’m not saying it was right, what you did. I’m not saying it was wrong, either. I’m just saying that the world is more complicated than most people want to believe.”

They ate together in silence for a while, sharing the simple meal that Kathleen had prepared. It was the first food Mary had tasted in weeks that carried the flavour of kindness rather than duty or punishment.

"Do you hate me?" Mary asked eventually.

Kathleen considered the question while she carefully wrapped the remaining bread for Mary to save for later. “No,” she said finally. I don’t hate you. I don’t love you either, I don’t know you well enough for that. But I understand you, I think. I understand what it’s like to be pushed so far by cruelty and injustice that you start looking for ways to push back.”

“I murdered thirty-seven people.”

“Yes, you did. And some of them probably deserved it, and some of them probably didn’t, and most of them probably fell somewhere in between like the rest of us.” Kathleen stood up, smoothing her skirts with work-worn hands. “The question isn’t whether what you did was right or wrong, that’s for God to judge. The question is what you do with whatever time you have left.”

After she left, Mary found herself thinking about Kathleen’s words. What did one do with three weeks of life when death was a certainty and redemption seemed impossible? How did someone like her, someone who had been broken and remade into an instrument of death, find meaning in the final chapter of their story?

The answer came to her gradually, over the course of several sleepless nights. She could not undo what she had done, could not bring her victims back to life or erase the terror she had spread. But she could tell the truth, not just about her crimes, but about the forces that had shaped her, the system that had broken her, the creature that had fed on her brokenness.

Mary began to write, using paper and ink that Father O'Malley brought her despite his theological struggles with her case. She wrote about her childhood in the cottage with the leaking roof, about the beatings and the hunger and the constant fear that had been her earliest education. She wrote about Padraig's attack and the moment when she discovered what she was capable of, about the years of killing her own family while their ghosts watched in sad resignation.

But she also wrote about An Dubhán, the ancient thing that had found her in her desperation and offered her power in exchange for becoming its instrument. She described how it had fed on death and terror, how it had gradually consumed her humanity until she became little more than a sophisticated weapon aimed at targets it selected.

The manuscript grew longer with each passing day, becoming not just a confession but a warning. Mary wrote about the signs to watch for, the way desperation could make someone vulnerable to forces that promised easy solutions to impossible problems. She wrote about the price of power, about how the pursuit of justice could become indistinguishable from the pursuit of revenge if one was not careful about the bargains one made.

On her final Sunday, Father O'Malley came to offer her last rites. He had wrestled with her case for weeks, consulting theologians and praying for guidance, but he had finally reached a conclusion that allowed him to do his duty as a priest.

"I cannot absolve you in the traditional sense," he told her, his young face grave with the weight of theological responsibility. "You have not shown the kind of repentance that the Church requires for full forgiveness. But I believe that your acceptance of responsibility, your willingness to face the consequences of your actions, represents a form of spiritual honesty that may be its own path to grace."

Mary knelt on the cold stone floor of her cell and accepted the sacrament, feeling neither saved nor damned but simply ready for whatever came next. When Father O'Malley had finished the ritual, she handed him the manuscript she had been working on for weeks.

"See that this gets to someone who might understand its importance," she told him. "Not the newspapers, they'll only sensationalise it. Find someone who studies such things, someone who might be able to warn others about the dangers of making bargains with forces they don't understand."

The priest took the manuscript with trembling hands, recognising its weight even without reading it. "I will," he promised.

The morning of Mary's execution dawned grey and cold, with a mist rising from the Liffey that made the world seem insubstantial, dreamlike. She had slept well for the first time in years, untroubled by nightmares or the whisper of ancient hungers in her mind. She felt clean, somehow, not forgiven, not redeemed, but honest in a way she had not been for decades.

As they led her to the gallows, Mary thought about the weight of stones that had shaped her life from the very beginning. The stones of her childhood cottage, the stone that had killed Padraig, the stone walls of Kilmainham Gaol that had held her in her final weeks. But now, as she climbed the wooden steps to meet her death, she felt as if the heaviest stones of all had finally been lifted from her shoulders.

The crowd that had gathered to witness her execution was large but strangely quiet. There were no jeers or calls for vengeance, only a hushed attention that suggested they understood they were witnessing something more complex than simple justice.

Mary looked out over the sea of faces and spoke her final words clearly, so that everyone present could hear them.

"I have killed thirty-seven people," she said. "I did it knowingly, willingly, and without the excuse of madness or passion. I deserve to die for my crimes, and I accept that judgment. But I hope that my death might serve as a warning, that desperation and pain can make anyone vulnerable to forces that promise power in exchange for humanity. Be careful what bargains you make when you are broken. The price may be higher than you imagine."

The executioner placed the hood over her head, and Mary's last conscious thought was of her family's ghosts, offering the forgiveness she had never thought to ask for. The rope tightened around her neck, and Mary Costello, murderer, victim, instrument of ancient hunger, and finally, perhaps, something approaching a human being again, stepped into whatever judgment awaited her on the other side of the veil.

The crowd dispersed slowly, thoughtfully, each person carrying with them the memory of a woman who had chosen truth over comfortable lies, who had faced her death with a dignity that somehow transcended the horror of her crimes. In the end, it was perhaps the most human thing she had done in twenty years.

Chapter Nine
The Other Side

Mary stood looking at her own corpse, and the strangest part was how unsurprising it felt.

Her body hung from the gallows in the yard of Kilmainham Gaol, neck bent at an unnatural angle, face hidden beneath the executioner's hood. The crowd was beginning to disperse, their voices muted by the morning mist that still clung to the grey stones of Dublin. But Mary herself, or whatever she had become, remained beside the scaffold, studying the shell she had just vacated with the same clinical detachment she had once brought to observing her victims' deaths.

She was translucent, she realised, able to see the details of the gallows' construction through her own ghostly hands. The sensation was not unlike looking through colored glass, except the glass was herself and the colour was the pale luminescence that seemed to emanate from her spirit form. She felt neither heavy nor light, neither hot nor cold, simply present in a way that defied the physical laws she had spent forty-three years learning to navigate.

"It's always disorienting the first time," a familiar voice said beside her.

Mary turned to see Padraig standing there, his ghostly form more solid and substantial than it had appeared during their confrontation at Blackwater Castle. He was watching the executioner cut down her body with an expression of profound sadness, as if her death represented not justice but merely another tragedy in an endless series of sorrows.

"You're still here," Mary observed. "I thought... When I chose to break free from An Dubhán, when you offered me forgiveness... I thought you would move on to whatever comes after."

""We've been waiting," Padraig replied, and Mary noticed the plural pronoun. Looking around, she could now see the rest of her family's ghosts, Cormac, Brigid, Seamus, even their mother, whom Mary had never met in life but recognised instantly by the resemblance she shared with her children. They stood in a loose circle around the gallows, their forms more vivid and present than any ghost had a right to be.

"Waiting for what?" Mary asked, though she suspected she already knew the answer.

"For you," her mother said, stepping forward with a grace that seemed to make the very air around her shimmer. "For our family to be complete again, for the circle to close that was broken so many years ago in that cottage beside the bog."

Mary stared at the woman who had died bringing her into the world, the woman whose death had marked Mary as cursed from her very first breath. Mairead Costello had been beautiful once; Mary could see that now she possessed the kind of fierce, determined beauty that could survive poverty and childbearing and the grinding hardships of Irish peasant life. But death had refined that beauty into something ethereal, luminous, touched with a sorrow that seemed to encompass all the world's suffering.

"I killed them," Mary said, gesturing toward her siblings' ghosts. "I murdered our father. I became something monstrous, something that fed on death and terror for twenty years. How can you speak of family, of completeness, when I destroyed everything that might have bound us together?"

"Because that's what family is," Seamus said, his ghostly voice carrying a gentleness that had been absent during his living years. "Not just the bonds of blood or affection, but the ties that connect us even when we've done everything possible to sever them. You killed us, yes. But you also freed us."

Mary blinked in confusion. "Freed you?"

"From the suffering that had consumed our lives," Cormac explained. "From the poverty and hunger and desperation that had turned us all into something less than human. When you struck me down at the bridge, I was already dying inside, consumed by bitterness and rage and the same capacity for cruelty that had infected our entire family. Death released me from that poison."

"And from the guilt," Brigid added softly. "The guilt of what we had done to you, how we had treated you, the role we had played in creating the person you became. In life, I was too proud and too angry to acknowledge my part in your transformation. In death, I've had decades to understand and accept responsibility for it."

Mary looked from one ghostly face to another, seeing in each a peace that had been entirely absent during their mortal years. Her family had found something in death that had eluded them in life, not just rest, but a genuine understanding of the forces that had shaped them all, the cycles of violence and desperation that had turned their cottage into a crucible of suffering.

"An Dubhán," she said suddenly, remembering the creature that had shaped so much of her existence. "Is it...?"

"Gone," her mother said firmly. ""Banished back to whatever darkness spawned it, cut off from the mortal world by your choice to embrace truth over power. It cannot touch you now, cannot touch any of us. The bargain you made with it died when you chose humanity over its promises."

The crowd around the gallows had mostly dispersed now, leaving only the official witnesses and the prison guards who would oversee the disposal of Mary's body. She watched with detached interest as they loaded her corpse onto a cart, preparing to take it to the unmarked grave that awaited criminals and paupers.

"What happens now?" Mary asked. "Do we... Move on? Is there a heaven or hell or judgment waiting for us?"

"That depends,"" Mairead replied, "on what you choose to do with your understanding."

""I don't understand."

Her mother smiled, and the expression transformed her entire ethereal being into something that seemed to glow with its own inner light. "You have a choice, daughter. The same choice that faces every soul at the moment of death, whether to carry forward the lessons learned in life, or to remain trapped by the patterns that defined your mortal existence."

"You could stay here," Padraig added. "Bound to the places where you committed your crimes, haunting the scenes of your murders as so many troubled spirits do. Many ghosts choose that path, endlessly reliving their worst moments, trapped in cycles of guilt and regret that serve no purpose but to perpetuate their own suffering."

"Or?" Mary asked, sensing that this was not the option her family was recommending.

"Or you could help us with the work we've been doing," Seamus said. "The work of watching over those who find themselves in the same desperate circumstances that once drove you to make such terrible bargains."

Mary felt a stirring of something she had not experienced in decades, curiosity, perhaps even hope. "What kind of work?"

"There are others,"" Cormac explained. "Living people who have been broken by circumstance, who find themselves vulnerable to the same forces that once claimed you. Desperate souls who might be tempted to make bargains with entities like An Dubhán, who might trade their humanity for power without understanding the true cost of such transactions."

"We watch them," Brigid said. "We try to guide them toward better choices, to show them alternatives to the darkness that seems so attractive when they're drowning in despair. It's not always successful, free will means people must ultimately choose their own paths, but sometimes we can make a difference."

Mary considered this, studying the faces of her family as they waited for her response. The idea of spending eternity trying to prevent others from making the mistakes she had made carried a kind of poetic justice that appealed to her. But more than that, it offered something she had never expected to find in death, purpose, meaning, a way to transform the hard-earned wisdom of her suffering into something that might actually help others.

"You would want me to work with you?" she asked. "After everything I've done, after all the pain I've caused?"

"Especially because of everything you've done," Mairead said gently. "Who is better to recognise the signs of someone being tempted by ancient hungers than the person who spent twenty years serving such a creature? Who better to warn others about the price of power than someone who paid it in full?"

Mary looked one last time at her body as the cart carrying it rumbled through the prison gates. That physical form had been the instrument of so much death, the vessel for so much cruelty and calculation. But it had also been the means by which she had finally found her way back to something approaching humanity, the tool through which she had chosen truth over comfortable lies.

"Yes," she said, the word carrying across the ethereal plane with a resonance that seemed to make the very air shimmer. "Yes, I'll help. I'll do whatever I can to keep others from following the path I chose."

Her family's ghosts smiled in unison, their forms growing brighter and more substantial as Mary joined their circle. She could feel something changing within her, a sense of connection and purpose that she had never experienced in life. The weight that had pressed down on her for so long, the weight of secrets, of guilt, of choices that could never be undone, was still there, but it had been transformed into something bearable, even meaningful.

"There's someone we need to help," Padraig said, his voice carrying new urgency. "A young man in Belfast, a dock worker whose family was killed in a fire started by his English supervisor's negligence. He's been approached by something old and hungry, something that promises him the power to take revenge on those responsible."

Mary felt a familiar chill, recognising the pattern even in this new form of existence. "How long do we have?"

"Not long," Seamus replied. "But perhaps long enough, if we move quickly and if you can remember exactly what it felt like when An Dubhán first whispered in your ear."

Mary nodded, feeling purpose crystallise within her ghostly form like ice forming on a winter pond. She had spent her life becoming a weapon of death and terror. Now, perhaps, she could spend whatever came after life becoming something else entirely, a shield, a warning, a voice of hard-earned wisdom in the darkness where desperate souls searched for easy answers to impossible questions.

The work would be difficult, possibly endless, certainly thankless. But as Mary felt herself beginning to fade from the physical world and move into whatever realm existed between life and final judgment, she found herself genuinely eager to begin.

She had been broken by circumstance and remade by ancient hungers into something monstrous. Now she would see if she could be remade once more, this time by choice, by purpose, by the hope that even the deepest darkness could serve some greater light.

The circle of her family's love closed around her, and Mary Costello stepped forward into her afterlife, carrying with her everything she had learned about the price of power and the possibility of redemption.

Chapter Ten
The Deception Unveiled

The young dock worker in Belfast was already dead by the time Mary and her family's ghosts arrived.

His body hung from a rope in his squalid tenement room, his face purple and swollen, his eyes bulging with the final terror of a man who had realised too late that he had been deceived. On the table beside his corpse lay a suicide note written in a shaking hand: "I cannot live with what I have become. God forgive me for the bargain I made.""

Mary stared at the scene, confusion and growing dread warring in her ethereal consciousness. They had rushed here with such urgency, her family speaking of the desperate need to save this young man from making the same mistake she had made decades ago. But they were too late, or were they?

"Strange," Padraig mused, his ghostly form circling the body with predatory interest. "We arrived exactly when we said we would, didn't we? Almost as if we knew precisely when young Thomas here would reach his breaking point."

Something cold that had nothing to do with her ghostly nature crawled up Mary's spine. There was something different about her brother's voice, something she hadn't noticed before in the overwhelming emotion of their reunion. It carried an undertone of satisfaction, of hunger fed rather than purpose thwarted.

"What do you mean?" Mary asked, though she was beginning to suspect she didn't want to know the answer.

"Oh, sister," Brigid laughed, and the sound was like breaking glass in a cathedral. "Sweet, naive Mary. Did you really think we spent all those years standing around your cottage out of some noble desire for justice? Did you imagine we were content to simply watch while you built your career as Ireland's most accomplished murderess?"

Mary felt her ghostly form beginning to tremble as understanding dawned like a sickly sunrise. "You were feeding. You were feeding on the deaths, just like An Dubhán."

"Feeding, yes," Cormac confirmed, his form beginning to shift and blur around the edges, becoming something less human and more primordial. "But not like that ancient thing you served so faithfully. We were feeding on something much more refined, much more... Personal."

The cottage materialised around them suddenly, not the stone hovel of Mary's childhood, but a twisted version of it, its walls weeping blood and its roof open to a sky that burned with unholy fire. They were no longer in Belfast, Mary realised. They were somewhere else entirely, somewhere that existed between the world of the living and whatever lay beyond death.

"Welcome home, daughter," Seamus said, his voice carrying the same cruel authority it had held in life but magnified a thousandfold. “Welcome to the place we built from your guilt, your desperate need for forgiveness, your pathetic desire to believe that family could mean something more than blood and violence and the endless cycle of hurt begetting hurt.”

Mary tried to flee, to return to the physical world or move forward into whatever judgment awaited her, but found herself trapped within the cottage’s bleeding walls. Her family’s ghosts surrounded her now, their forms revealing themselves to be something far more terrible than the spirits of murdered victims.

“You’re not my family,” Mary whispered, the truth cutting through her like a blade forged from her own despair. “You never were my family. What are you?”

“We are what your guilt created,” Mairead said, her beautiful face melting into something with too many eyes and teeth like broken stars. “We are the punishment you inflicted upon yourself, given form and substance by decades of self-recrimination and desperate longing for redemption that could never come.”

The creature that had worn her mother’s face leaned closer, its breath carrying the scent of grave dirt and rotting flowers. “You killed your real family, Mary. Murdered them in fits of rage and desperation and then spent years telling yourself it was justified, that they deserved what you gave them. But deep in your heart, you knew the truth, you were a monster who had destroyed the only people who might have loved you, given the chance.”

“So you created us,” the thing that had been Padraig continued. "Manifestations of your own guilt and need, spirits born from your desperate desire to believe that somewhere, somehow, your victims had found peace and could offer you forgiveness. We became real because you needed us to be real, substantial because your guilt was substantial enough to give us form."

Mary sank to her knees on the cottage's blood-soaked floor, understanding flooding through her like poison through veins. Every moment of peace she had felt since her execution, every surge of hope and purpose, every warm glow of familial acceptance, all of it had been a lie she had told herself, a fantasy constructed from her own desperate need to believe that redemption was possible.

"The young man in Belfast," she gasped. "Did we really fail to save him, or...?"

"Oh, we saved him beautifully," Brigid laughed, her form now a writhing mass of shadow and malice. "Saved him from a life of guilt and suffering and the slow poison of revenge. We whispered to him in his darkest moments, convinced him that the bargain he had made with forces beyond his understanding could never be undone, that suicide was his only escape from what he had become. We fed on his despair just as we fed on yours, growing stronger with each moment of anguish we inspired."

The cottage around them pulsed like a living heart, its walls expanding and contracting with each breath of Mary's horror. She understood now that this place was not a prison but a digestive organ, a spiritual stomach where her false family could slowly consume everything that remained of her essence.

"But why?" Mary asked, her voice barely a whisper. "Why go through such an elaborate deception? Why not simply devour me the moment I die?"

"Because guilt taken freely is so much more nourishing than guilt imposed by force," the creature wearing Seamus's face explained. "When you chose to 'redeem' yourself, when you embraced what you thought was your family's forgiveness and dedicated your afterlife to helping others, you were seasoning yourself for us. Each moment of hope made your eventual despair more exquisite, each surge of purpose made your final understanding of meaninglessness more delicious.""

Mary felt herself beginning to fade, her ghostly form growing translucent as the creatures that had masqueraded as her family began to feed in earnest. But even as her essence was being consumed, even as she felt herself dissolving into the spiritual equivalent of digestive acids, a part of her mind remained clear and calculating.

These things had made a mistake. In their eagerness to savour her despair, to feed on the exquisite anguish of her final understanding, they had revealed too much about their nature. They were not her family's ghosts, they never had been. They were parasitic entities that fed on guilt and self-recrimination, creatures that required their victims' willing participation in their own destruction.

But Mary had spent twenty years learning to see through deceptions, to recognise when she was being manipulated by forces that promised more than they intended to deliver. An Dubhán had taught her that lesson, even if the ancient creature had ultimately fallen victim to the same patterns it had tried to exploit.

"You're right," Mary said suddenly, her voice cutting through the creatures' feeding frenzy like a sword through silk. “I did kill my family. I murdered them in cold blood, without remorse, without the excuse of madness or passion. I destroyed the only people who might have loved me, and I did it because it was easier than trying to find another way to survive.”

The parasitic entities paused in their consumption, sensing something changing in their prey but not yet understanding what it meant.

“I became a monster,” Mary continued, her form growing slightly more solid as she spoke. “I served an ancient evil, murdered dozens of innocent people, spread terror throughout Ireland for my own profit and satisfaction. I am guilty of crimes so terrible that no earthly court could have imposed adequate punishment for them.”

“Yes,” the thing that had worn Mairead’s face hissed with satisfaction. “Yes, embrace your guilt, feed our hunger with your despair...x ”

xxxxxxxxxxxx“But I am not guilty of being deceived by you,” Mary said, and her voice now carried an authority that made the cottage’s walls tremble. “I am not guilty of hoping for redemption, of wanting to believe that even someone like me might find a way to atone for what I’ve done. That hope was not a weakness, it was the last human thing left in me, and you have no right to feed on it.”

The creatures recoiled as if struck, their false forms wavering as Mary’s understanding solidified into something approaching power. She was still trapped within their spiritual digestive chamber, still being slowly consumed by their alien hunger, but she was no longer a willing participant in her own destruction.

"My guilt is my own," Mary declared, rising to her feet on the cottage's blood-soaked floor. "My crimes are my responsibility, my punishment is mine to bear. But my hope, pathetic and misguided though it may have been, belongs to me, not to you. And I will not let you take it from me."

The false cottage began to shake, its blood-weeping walls cracking as the parasitic entities' feeding was disrupted by their prey's sudden resistance. Mary could feel her essence still being drawn from her, but the process was no longer smooth and inevitable. She was fighting back, asserting her right to her own spiritual destruction rather than allowing these creatures to orchestrate it for their nourishment.

""You cannot resist us," the thing that had been Cormac snarled, its form now revealed as a writhing mass of spiritual hunger and predatory need. "You are already dead, already guilty, already ours to consume. Your resistance only prolongs your suffering."

"Perhaps," Mary agreed. "But it's my suffering now, isn't it? My choice to resist, my decision to fight, my right to go into whatever darkness awaits me on my own terms rather than yours."

The cottage was collapsing around them now, its false walls crumbling like dreams in the harsh light of morning. But Mary was not trying to escape, she understood that these creatures were part of her now, born from her guilt and sustained by her need for punishment. She could not banish them or flee from them any more than she could flee from her own shadow.

But she could choose how they would consume her. She could decide whether to go down fighting or to surrender meekly to their alien hunger. And after everything she had done, after all the choices she had made in service to powers greater than herself, Mary Costello was finally ready to make a choice that was entirely her own.

The battle for what remained of her soul had begun, and for the first time since her death, Mary felt something approaching peace. Not because she expected to win, she understood that victory, in any meaningful sense, was probably impossible. But because she was finally, truly fighting for herself rather than serving the agenda of something else.

The rage that filled Mary was unlike anything she had ever experienced, even during her most violent moments as a living woman. It was not the cold, calculating fury that had driven her to murder her siblings, nor the professional detachment that had guided her hand as Catherine Blackthorne. This was something pure and primal, a spiritual fire that burned away twenty years of carefully constructed guilt and self-recrimination like morning mist before the sun.

"You dare," she snarled, her ghostly form blazing with a light that made the parasitic creat`ures shriek and recoil. "You dare wear their faces, speak with their voices, offer me the forgiveness that should have been theirs to give or withhold?"

The cottage around them began to burn, not with earthly flames, but with the incandescent fury of a soul that had finally, truly, been pushed too far. Mary's rage was consuming the very spiritual architecture that the creatures had built from her guilt, reducing their feeding chamber to ash and memory.

"I killed them!" Mary roared, her voice shaking the foundations of whatever realm contained them. I murdered Padraig and Cormac and Brigid and Seamus! I watched the life drain from their eyes, felt their blood on my hands, and buried their bodies in unmarked graves! That guilt is MINE! Those deaths are MY responsibility! You have no right to them, no claim to the remorse they earned through their suffering!"

The thing that had worn Mairead's face writhed in agony as Mary's fury struck it like a physical blow. "Your guilt feeds us," it gasped, its false form dissolving into something that resembled melting wax. "Your self-hatred sustains us. Without that nourishment, we cannot"

"Then starve," Mary said, her words carrying the finality of a judge' sentence. "Starve and fade and return to whatever emptiness spawned you. I withdraw my guilt from your table. I reclaim my crimes as my own."

But even as she spoke, Mary understood that rage alone would not be enough to free her from these creatures. They were not external enemies she could fight with fury and determination, they were part of her spiritual anatomy now, born from psychological needs that had shaped her since childhood. To truly banish them, she would need to do something far more difficult than simply being angry.

She would need to forgive herself.

The realization stopped her cold, draining the fire from her ghostly form and leaving her standing in the ruins of the false cottage with nothing but the weight of her own understanding. The parasitic entities sensed the change immediately, their forms beginning to solidify again as they prepared to resume their feeding.

"Yes," the creature that had been Cormac hissed with renewed hunger. "You see it now, don't you? The impossible task that faces you. How do you forgive someone who has done what you have done? How do you grant yourself the mercy you denied to so many others?"

Mary stared at the writhing things that surrounded her, seeing them clearly for what they were, manifestations of her own inability to live with what she had become. They had no independent existence beyond her need to punish herself, no substance beyond the guilt she had fed them for decades.

"I don't know," she admitted, her voice quiet but steady. "I don't know how to forgive myself for what I've done. I don't know if such forgiveness is even possible, or if I have the right to grant it to myself."

The creatures pressed closer, sensing victory, their forms growing more solid and predatory. "Then you are ours," the false Brigid whispered. "Ours to consume slowly, eternally, as you devour yourself from within with guilt that can never be resolved."

"Perhaps," Mary agreed. "But if I am to be consumed, it will be by my own choices, not by your manipulation of them."

She closed her eyes and tried to remember her real family, not as the idealised spirits she had created from her guilt, but as they had actually been. Padraig, cruel and predatory but also broken by the same poverty and desperation that had shaped them all. Cormac, violent and bitter but also frightened, lashing out at the world that had given him so few options. Brigid, sharp-tongued and hateful, but also trying desperately to survive in circumstances that offered little hope for anything better.

And Seamus, their father, brutal and neglectful, yes, but also a man who had watched his dreams crumble, who had seen his children hungry and his wife dead and had found no way to bear that weight except through drink and violence.

They had been flawed, damaged people who had done terrible things to a child who deserved better. But they had also been human beings, trapped in cycles of poverty and desperation that had offered them few chances for anything resembling redemption.

Mary had killed them not out of noble justice but out of rage and fear and the simple, terrible need to make the pain stop. She had taken their lives not because she was a force of righteous vengeance but because she was a damaged child who had learned that violence was the only language her world understood.

“I'm sorry,”" she whispered, and the words were addressed not to the parasitic creatures that surrounded her but to the memories of her real family. “I’m sorry I killed you. I’m sorry I never gave you the chance to grow beyond what poverty and suffering had made you. I'm sorry I became something even worse than what you were.”

The creatures recoiled as if struck, their forms wavering as Mary’s genuine remorse, not the guilty self-flagellation they had been feeding on, but actual sorrow for lives cut short, disrupted their spiritual digestion.

"But I'm also sorry for what you did to me," Mary continued, her voice growing stronger. "Sorry that you beat me and starved me and taught me that love was something that had to be taken by force. Sorry that you created the circumstances that made me vulnerable to An Dubhán's influence, that gave me the skills I would later use to become a killer."

The false cottage was dissolving around them now, its blood-soaked walls crumbling as Mary spoke truths that the parasitic entities could not process or digest.

"We were all victims," Mary said, understanding flooding through her like clean water washing away decades of accumulated filth. "Victims of poverty, of a system that ground Irish families into dust, of circumstances that offered us violence or surrender as our only choices. That doesn't excuse what any of us did, not your cruelty to me, not my murders of you, not the twenty years I spent serving ancient hungers. But it explains it. It makes it human rather than simply monstrous.""

The creatures were fading now, their forms becoming translucent as they lost their grip on Mary's spiritual essence. They had been built from guilt and self-hatred, sustained by her need to punish herself for crimes that seemed to demand eternal torment. But they could not survive in the presence of genuine understanding, of the kind of clear-eyed acceptance that saw both crime and circumstance, both responsibility and context.

"I cannot forgive myself completely," Mary said as the last of the false spirits dissolved into memory and shadow. "What I did was too terrible, too calculated, too deliberately chosen to ever be fully absolved. But I can stop feeding my guilt like a pet that grows larger and more demanding with each meal."

She stood alone now in a space that was neither the physical world nor the false cottage, but something that might have been the quiet place between judgment and whatever came after. The parasitic entities were gone, banished not by rage or denial but by the simple act of seeing them clearly and choosing not to sustain them with her own self-destruction.

Mary felt lighter somehow, as if spiritual weights she had carried for decades had finally been set down. Not forgotten, she would carry the memory of her crimes forever, but no longer the defining feature of her existence. She was guilty, yes. But she was also human, and humanity included the possibility of growth, of understanding, of moving forward rather than being forever trapped in the worst moments of one's past.

The question now was what came next. She had escaped the parasitic spirits born from her own guilt, but that did not mean she had escaped judgment entirely. Somewhere beyond this quiet place, she sensed, waited whatever accounting the universe demanded from souls who had chosen power over humanity, who had served ancient hungers rather than their own conscience.

But for the first time since she had struck Padraig with that stone in the grove, Mary felt ready to face that judgment, not as a victim of her circumstances or a servant of alien wills, but as Mary Costello, a woman who had made terrible choices and was prepared to accept the consequences of them.

Chapter Eleven
The Devil's Bargain

The voice that spoke to Mary in the quiet space between judgments was nothing like An Dubhán's whispered seductions. This was authority incarnate, power so vast and ancient that it made the bog creature seem like a mewling child by comparison. When it spoke, reality itself seemed to bend and reshape around the weight of its words.

"Mary Costello,"" it said, and her name in that voice carried the sound of empires falling and worlds ending. "How refreshing to find a soul that has managed to escape the tedious cycle of guilt and self-recrimination. So few manage to see their parasites for what they truly are."

Mary turned toward the voice, though turning had no meaning in this placeless place. What she saw defied description, not because it was incomprehensible, but because it was too perfectly comprehensible, too exactly what every human instinct recognised as the source of all temptation and corruption. If An Dubhán had been hunger given form, this was ambition made manifest, the crystallized essence of every choice that sacrificed conscience for power.

"You're the Devil," Mary said, and it was not a question.

"One of many names I've worn," the entity replied, its form shifting between shapes that might have been beautiful, terrible, or simply inevitable. “Lucifer, Satan, the Adversary, all masks for what I truly am. I am the voice that whispers in the darkness when mortals grow tired of being powerless. I am the option that presents itself when every other choice leads to suffering.”

Mary felt no fear in the presence of this ultimate evil, which surprised her. Perhaps death had burned away her capacity for such emotions, or perhaps she had simply seen too much to be impressed by even the most grandiose displays of malevolence.

“What do you want?” she asked.

“To offer you something that very few souls have ever been granted,” the Devil replied, circling her with movements that suggested a predator evaluating prey. “A chance to return to life, to reclaim flesh and blood and breath, to walk the world again with all the power and knowledge you accumulated during your first existence.”

Mary felt something stir within her ghostly essence, not hope, exactly, but a hunger she had thought extinguished by death and revelation. “In exchange for what?”

“Service, naturally,” the Devil said with what might have been amusement. “But not the crude servitude you offered to that ancient bog-thing. I require agents of sophistication, souls who understand that true power comes not from random violence but from systematic corruption of everything that humans hold sacred.”

The space around them began to shift and change, revealing visions of what such service might entail. Mary saw herself returned to flesh, young and beautiful again, moving through the world with resources and influence beyond anything Catherine Blackthorne had possessed. She saw herself in positions of power, advisor to kings, confidante to bishops, the hidden hand that guided nations toward decisions that would damn millions of souls.

"You offer me life," Mary said, watching the visions with the same clinical interest she had once brought to studying potential victims. "But what kind of life? What would I become?"

"You would become what you were always meant to be," the Devil replied, his voice carrying seductive certainty. "Not a crude killer serving an ancient appetite, but an artist of damnation, a craftsman of spiritual corruption. You would be my left hand in the world, charged with creating the circumstances that drive others to make the same choices you once made."

Mary saw more visions, herself establishing networks of desperation and temptation, creating the conditions that would make ordinary people vulnerable to the kinds of bargains she had once accepted. She would not kill with poison or blade, but with systems and institutions that slowly drained hope from the world until darkness seemed like the only refuge.

"I would be creating more people like myself," she observed.

"Exactly," the Devil confirmed. "You understand the process intimately, the precise combination of suffering and opportunity that transforms a victim into a predator. Who better to orchestrate such transformations on a grand scale?"

The offer hung in the void between them like a star balanced on the edge of collapse. Mary could feel the power that accompanied it, the promise of influence that would dwarf anything she had achieved in her mortal existence. She would be returned to life not as a peasant girl or even as a lady of quality, but as something approaching a force of nature, beautiful, wealthy, connected, capable of reshaping the world according to her vision.

"And if I refuse?" she asked, though she was surprised to find herself seriously considering acceptance.

"Then you continue forward to whatever judgment awaits you," the Devil said with apparent indifference. "Perhaps eternal punishment for your crimes, perhaps simple dissolution into the void that preceded your existence. I care little either way, there are always other souls willing to accept what you might reject."

Mary closed her eyes and tried to think clearly about the choice before her. She had just freed herself from parasitic entities that had fed on her guilt and self-recrimination. She had found a kind of peace in accepting responsibility for her actions while refusing to let that responsibility consume her entirely. She had been prepared to face whatever final judgment awaited her with something approaching dignity.

But the Devil's offer represented something she had never expected to encounter, a chance to return to the game, to reclaim agency and power in a world that had always denied both to people like her. Not as a servant this time, but as a partner, an architect of the very systems that created the suffering she had once experienced.

"I accept," Mary said, the words leaving her spiritual form before she had fully consciously decided to speak them.

The Devil's laughter was like the sound of everything beautiful in the world being ground to dust beneath the wheel of necessity. "Of course you do," he said with satisfaction. "You were never truly repentant, were you, Mary Costello? Oh, you felt sorry for the pain you caused, regretted the waste and inefficiency of your methods. But you never actually wished you had chosen differently, never genuinely desired to have been a good person living a small, quiet life."

Mary felt the truth of his words settling into her consciousness like stones into deep water. Her moment of clarity in the previous chapter had freed her from the guilt-feeding parasites, but it had not changed her fundamental nature. She was still the woman who had chosen power over mercy, efficiency over conscience, personal agency over moral constraint.

"You're right," she admitted. "Given the same circumstances, the same choices, I would make the same decisions again. Not because they were right, but because they were mine."

"And that, my dear Mary, is why you are so perfectly suited for what I have in mind," the Devil said, extending what might have been a hand toward her. "Shall we begin your resurrection?"

Mary reached out to clasp the offered appendage, feeling reality begin to shift and reform around her as the bargain was sealed. She was returning to life, but not to the life she had known. She was being reborn as something new, something designed from the ground up to serve purposes that would make her previous crimes seem like the fumbling experiments of an enthusiastic amateur.

"What will my name be?" she asked as flesh began to form around her spiritual essence like clay around an armature.

"Whatever you choose," the Devil replied. "Though I suspect you'll find that names matter less than the roles you inhabit, the positions you claim, the influence you wield. You are becoming something beyond individual identity, you are becoming a function of corruption itself."

Mary felt her heart begin to beat again, felt breath fill lungs that had been dust and ash, felt the familiar weight of physical existence settling around her like a comfortable coat. But she also felt something else, a connection to vast networks of power and influence, knowledge flowing into her mind about how the world truly worked, who really made the decisions that shaped nations and faiths and the dreams of ordinary people.

"What is my first assignment?" she asked, her voice carrying through vocal cords that had never existed before this moment.

"Patience," the Devil said with amusement. "First, you must be properly introduced to the world that awaits you. There is much to learn about how power truly operates in this age of reason and revolution. The crude methods of your first life would be woefully inadequate for what I have planned."

Mary nodded, feeling anticipation building in her newly restored chest. She had served ancient hunger and learned its limitations. She had experienced genuine remorse and discovered her powerlessness. Now she would serve ultimate corruption and explore its possibilities.

She was no longer Mary Costello, Irish peasant and failed seeker of redemption. She was something new, something unprecedented, something that would reshape the world according to visions that no mortal mind could fully comprehend.

The Devil's bloody work was about to begin in earnest, and Mary found herself eager to discover just how much damnation one resurrected soul could accomplish when given the proper resources and motivation.

Her second life was beginning, and it would make her first existence look like the innocent play of children compared to the sophisticated artistry of corruption she was about to unleash upon the world.

Chapter Twelve
Bloody Mary

The woman who emerged from the shadows of St. Bartholomew's Cathedral in London bore no resemblance to the peasant girl who had died on a Dublin gallows three months earlier. Lady Margaret Sanguinaire was tall and elegant, with auburn hair that caught light like liquid copper and eyes the coour of old blood. Her dress was cut from the finest silk, her jewellery spoke of wealth accumulated across generations, and her accent carried the refined cadences of someone educated in the best finishing schools of Europe.

But it was not her beauty or her obvious prosperity that made men step aside when she passed, that made servants hurry to fulfil her slightest request, that made even hardened London criminals cross themselves when they heard her name whispered in taverns and gaming hells. It was something else entirely, an aura of controlled danger that suggested she could smile while ordering your death, that she understood exactly how much pain a human soul could endure before it finally broke.

Lady Sanguinaire had appeared in London society six weeks after Mary Costello's execution, armed with impeccable credentials that traced her lineage back to Norman nobles and her fortune to successful investments in the slave plantations of Jamaica. She had rented a magnificent house in Mayfair, staffed it with servants who asked no questions and remembered nothing inconvenient, and begun the slow work of infiltrating the networks of power that controlled the British Empire.

The Devil had been as good as his word. The knowledge he had poured into her resurrected mind was vast and sophisticated, encompassing not just the crude techniques of murder and manipulation she had learned in her first life, but the subtler arts of corruption that could destroy souls without ever shedding blood. She understood now how to turn virtue into vice, how to make men betray their deepest principles while believing themselves to be acting nobly, how to create systems of seemingly benevolent oppression that would damn generations yet unborn.

But perhaps most importantly, she understood patience. Where Mary Costello had been driven by rage and desperation to seek immediate solutions to her problems, Lady Sanguinaire could afford to think in decades, in centuries, in the kind of generational schemes that reshaped entire civilisations. She was no longer an individual seeking revenge or profit, she was an agent of ultimate corruption, charged with planting seeds that would bloom into damnation long after her current identity had been discarded and forgotten.

Her first target was Sir Edmund Harwick, the prosecutor who had argued so eloquently for her execution at the trial of Mary Costello. She found him in his club on a foggy November evening, celebrating his recent appointment to the Queen's Counsel with a group of his legal colleagues. He was a man intoxicated by his own righteousness, convinced that his prosecution of the infamous murderess had been a triumph of justice over evil.

Lady Sanguinaire approached him with the perfect combination of deference and intrigue, introducing herself as a woman with certain legal difficulties that might benefit from his expertise. Sir Edmund was initially reluctant, he had no need of additional income, and his recent fame had brought him cases more prestigious than anything a colonial widow might offer. But there was something about Lady Sanguinaire that captured his attention, a quality that made him want to be near her, to bask in whatever dark radiance she carried.

"I find myself in possession of certain documents," she said, her voice low and intimate despite the public setting. "Papers that reveal the involvement of highly placed individuals in... Unseemly activities. The kind of activities that could destroy reputations, topple governments, reshape the very foundations of our society."

Sir Edmund's eyes gleamed with interest despite himself. He was an ambitious man, and ambition always responded to the promise of leverage over the powerful.

"What sort of activities?" he asked, leaning closer to hear her reply.

"The slave trade, primarily," Lady Sanguinaire replied, watching his face carefully. "But not the legal variety that has made so many fortunes for good English families. I speak of arrangements that continued after Parliament banned the practice of ships that sailed under false flags, of prominent abolitionists who profited from the very system they publicly condemned."

She produced a leather portfolio from her reticule, allowing Sir Edmund to glimpse documents that appeared to bear official seals and signatures he recognised. The papers were forgeries, of course, but forgeries so perfect that they would fool any expert examination. The Devil's resources extended far beyond what Mary Costello could ever have imagined.

"These documents could destroy half the House of Lords," Sir Edmund breathed, his prosecutor's mind already calculating the implications. "The scandal would be unprecedented. The government would fall, fortunes would be lost, reputations built over generations would crumble to dust."

"Precisely," Lady Sanguinaire agreed. "The question is what should be done with such explosive information. Should it be revealed for the good of the public, regardless of the chaos that would follow? Or should it be... Managed... In a way that serves justice while preserving the stability that our society requires?"

Sir Edmund stared at the documents with the fascination of a moth drawn to flame. He understood what she was truly offering, not just information, but the power to decide how that information would be used. He could expose the guilty and watch the empire convulse with scandal, or he could use the threat of exposure to reshape the government according to his own vision of justice.

"What do you want in return for this intelligence?" he asked, though he suspected he already knew the answer would be more complex than simple payment.

"Partnership," Lady Sanguinaire replied. "I am a woman, Sir Edmund, which limits my ability to act directly in matters of law and politics. But you are a man of proven capability, someone who has already demonstrated your commitment to seeing justice done regardless of the cost. Together, we could ensure that these revelations serve the cause of righteousness rather than mere destruction."

Over the following weeks, Sir Edmund found himself drawn deeper into Lady Sanguinaire's web of promises and implications. She provided him with document after document, each one more damaging than the last, each one offering him greater leverage over the powerful men who had previously been beyond his reach. But she also provided him with something else, a philosophy of justice that justified increasingly extreme measures in service of righteous goals.

"Sometimes," she would tell him as they reviewed evidence of corruption in the highest levels of government, "mercy becomes complicity. Sometimes the only way to truly serve justice is to become more ruthless than the criminals we pursue."

Sir Edmund found himself nodding along to her arguments, found himself agreeing that conventional legal procedures were inadequate for dealing with crimes of such magnitude. When Lady Sanguinaire suggested that certain key witnesses might need to be "protected" from those who would silence them, he readily agreed to arrangements that placed them under her personal supervision. When she recommended that some of the evidence be obtained through methods that might not pass strict legal scrutiny, he chose to look the other way in service of the greater good.

He did not realise that the witnesses were being systematically corrupted rather than protected, that Lady Sanguinaire was teaching them to lie convincingly rather than helping them tell the truth. He did not understand that the evidence she provided was being carefully curated to serve her purposes rather than those of justice. He believed himself to be a righteous man using questionable methods for noble ends, never suspecting that he was being systematically transformed into an instrument of the very corruption he thought he was fighting.

The scandal, when it finally broke, was everything Lady Sanguinaire had promised. Half of Parliament was implicated in illegal slave trading, prominent abolitionists were revealed as hypocrites who had profited from human misery while publicly condemning it, and the government collapsed amid accusations and counter-accusations that seemed to implicate nearly everyone in positions of power.

But the chaos that followed was not the cleansing fire of justice that Sir Edmund had expected. Instead, it was something darker and more destructive, a breakdown of trust in all institutions, a cynical assumption that everyone was corrupt and that moral authority was merely a mask worn by those who sought to exploit the gullible. The revelations did not create a better world; they created a world where virtue itself became suspect, where the very concept of righteousness was poisoned by the understanding that it had so often been used as a cover for exploitation.

Sir Edmund found himself at the centre of the storm, hailed as a hero by some and condemned as a destroyer by others. But more troubling than either praise or blame was his growing understanding of what he had become. In his pursuit of justice through Lady Sanguinaire's methods, he had learned to lie, to manipulate, to sacrifice innocent people for strategic advantage. He had told himself that these were necessary evils in the service of a greater good, but he could no longer ignore the fact that evil was exactly what they were.

The night he finally confronted Lady Sanguinaire with his doubts, she received him in the library of her Mayfair house with the same elegant composure she had shown during their first meeting. She listened to his accusations and self-recriminations with apparent sympathy, nodding along as he explained how their partnership had transformed him into something he could barely recognize.

"You're right, of course," she said when he had finished. "You have become something different from what you were. The question is whether you have become something better or something worse."

"How can you ask that?" Sir Edmund demanded. "Look at what we've done! Look at the chaos we've unleashed! I set out to serve justice and ended up destroying the very foundations of the system I swore to uphold!"

Lady Sanguinaire smiled, and in that expression, Sir Edmund finally saw something of what she truly was, not a woman seeking justice through questionable means, but a predator who had been playing with her prey all along.

"But did the system deserve to be upheld?" she asked gently. "Was the stability you've destroyed really worth preserving, or was it simply a comfortable lie that allowed terrible injustices to continue unchallenged? You have done something that no conventional prosecutor could have achieved, you have forced an entire empire to confront the contradictions between its stated values and its actual practices."

Sir Edmund stared at her, understanding finally dawning. "You planned this. All of it. The documents, the revelations, the chaos that followed, you orchestrated everything."

"I provided opportunities," Lady Sanguinaire corrected. "You made the choices. Every decision to bend the rules, every compromise with your principles, every moment when you chose efficiency over ethics, those were your choices, Sir Edmund. I merely created the circumstances that revealed what kind of man you truly were when tested."

The realisation broke something in Sir Edmund's mind. He had always believed himself to be fundamentally good, someone who might make mistakes but who would never willingly serve evil. To discover that he had been manipulated into betraying everything he claimed to believe was devastating enough. But to understand that the manipulation had only succeeded because something in his nature had been eager to be corrupted, that was unbearable.

He left Lady Sanguinaire's house that night and walked directly to the Thames, where his body was found three days later, apparently having thrown himself from

Westminster Bridge in a fit of remorse and despair. The newspapers attributed his suicide to the strain of the massive corruption investigation he had led, never suspecting that his death was itself the final act in a drama of damnation orchestrated by forces beyond human understanding.

Lady Sanguinaire read the news of his death over breakfast, feeling the familiar satisfaction of work well done. Sir Edmund Harwick had been more than just a target for revenge, he had been a test case, an opportunity to refine the techniques the Devil had taught her. She had learned valuable lessons about the pace of corruption, about the importance of allowing victims to believe they were making their own choices, about the exquisite pleasure of watching supposedly righteous men discover their own capacity for evil.

The British Empire would recover from the scandal, of course. New politicians would rise to replace those who had fallen, and new systems would be established to prevent such corruption in the future. But the more serious damage had been done, the damage to faith in moral authority itself, the poisoning of the very concept of righteousness that would make future corruption easier to achieve and harder to recognise.

Lady Sanguinaire finished her breakfast and began planning her next project. There were so many institutions that needed corrupting, so many souls that could be led down the path of damnation through their own choices and desires. She had eternity to work with, and she was just beginning to understand the true scope of what the Devil's service could accomplish.

Mary Costello had been a crude killer who had served ancient hunger for twenty years. But Bloody Mary, as the whispers in London's underworld had begun to call her, was something far more dangerous. She was corruption incarnate, damnation wearing a beautiful face, the promise of easy solutions to impossible problems.

And she was just getting started.

Within a month of Sir Edmund's suicide, Lady Sanguinaire had disappeared from London society as mysteriously as she had arrived. The house in Mayfair was found empty, its servants vanished without trace, its elegant furnishings covered in dust as if they had been abandoned for years rather than days. Those who asked after her were told that Lady Sanguinaire had returned to her estates in Jamaica, though no ship's manifest recorded her departure and no plantation records bore her name.

The truth was far more complex. Mary had learned from the Devil that true corruption required constant reinvention, that staying too long in any single identity would limit her effectiveness. Sir Edmund's case had taught her valuable lessons, but it had also made her face too familiar to certain circles in London. It was time to become someone else, to find new hunting grounds where her methods could be refined and perfected.

She materialised in Dublin six weeks later as Sister Magdalene Caritas, a nun of unusual beauty and compelling presence who had come from Rome bearing credentials from the Vatican itself. Her mission, she explained to the local bishops, was to establish new charitable institutions that would address the lingering devastation caused by the recent famine. She spoke with passionate eloquence about the need to help Ireland's suffering masses, to create systems of aid that would prevent future disasters while addressing the spiritual as well as physical needs of the people.

The Catholic hierarchy in Ireland was initially suspicious, Rome rarely sent female emissaries on missions of such importance, and Sister Magdalene's youth and beauty seemed incongruous with the gravity of her supposed calling. But she carried letters of introduction signed by cardinals whose signatures were unquestionably authentic, and her knowledge of Church doctrine and administrative procedures was encyclopedic. More importantly, she brought with her promises of funding that could transform Ireland's charitable infrastructure overnight.

Within weeks of her arrival, Sister Magdalene had established herself at the centre of Dublin's religious and political circles. She met with bishops and politicians, with wealthy merchants and influential landowners, with anyone who might have the power to shape policy or allocate resources. Her proposals were ambitious but practical, workhouses that would provide not just shelter but education and vocational training, hospitals that would serve both the body and the soul, schools that would prepare Irish children for productive lives while ensuring their continued devotion to the faith.

But Sister Magdalene's vision of charity was subtly different from the conventional Christian understanding of mercy and compassion. Her institutions, she explained, would be designed to help people help themselves, to teach them that salvation required not just faith but active participation in their own moral and material improvement. Those who proved themselves worthy through hard work and submission to proper authority would receive increasing levels of support and opportunity. Those who failed to demonstrate such worthiness would find their assistance reduced or withdrawn entirely.

"Charity without accountability," she would tell her listeners with conviction that rang like bells in a cathedral, "is not mercy but cruelty. It teaches people to depend on others rather than developing their own capacity for righteousness. True Christian love requires that we help our brothers and sisters become the best versions of themselves, even when that requires difficult choices and painful lessons."

The theology was seductive because it contained elements of genuine truth. Self-reliance was indeed a virtue, accountability was important for moral development, and indiscriminate charity could sometimes enable destructive behaviours rather than correcting them. But Sister Magdalene's interpretation of these principles was carefully calibrated to serve darker purposes than those her listeners imagined.

Her first major project was the establishment of St. Bridget's Workhouse for Indigent Women, a facility ostensibly designed to provide shelter and vocational training for Dublin's female beggars and prostitutes. The building she selected was an imposing Gothic structure on the outskirts of the city, its high walls and narrow windows giving it the appearance of a convent crossed with a prison. She staffed it with nuns whose devotion was unquestionable but whose interpretation of Christian mercy had been subtly corrupted by her influence.

The women who entered St. Bridget's found themselves subject to a regime of moral education that was both rigorous and insidious. They were required to confess not just their sins but their sinful thoughts, to examine their consciences with a thoroughness that bordered on self-torture. They were taught that their poverty and degradation were not simply matters of unfortunate circumstance but reflections of their spiritual unworthiness, evidence of moral failings that required constant vigilance and self-denial to overcome.

Those who embraced this teaching, who demonstrated proper submission to the institution's authority and genuine remorse for their past failings, were rewarded with better food, more comfortable quarters, and opportunities to serve as supervisors over their fellow inmates. But those who questioned the system, who suggested that their circumstances might be due to forces beyond their control, or who failed to show adequate gratitude for the charity they received, found themselves subjected to increasingly harsh discipline designed to break their pride and teach them proper humility.

Sister Magdalene visited the workhouse regularly, moving through its corridors with the serene authority of someone whose every word carried the weight of divine approval. She would interview the women individually, listening to their confessions and complaints with apparent sympathy while carefully noting which inmates showed signs of dangerous independent thinking.

"Mary Sullivan,"" she said one afternoon to a young woman who had been brought to St. Bridget's after being found soliciting near the docks, "I understand you've been expressing doubts about our methods here. You've suggested to other women that perhaps their poverty is not entirely their fault, that society itself might bear some responsibility for their circumstances."'

Mary Sullivan was barely eighteen, with the kind of defiant beauty that poverty had not yet managed to crush entirely. She had been raised by a father who worked the docks when work was available and drank away his wages when it was not, and she had learned early that survival sometimes required making choices that proper society would condemn.

"I've said that some of the women here never had much choice in what they became," Mary replied, meeting Sister Magdalene's gaze with a boldness that would have been admirable in other circumstances. "When you're starving, and your children are crying for food, when landlords are demanding rent you can't pay, and there's no honest work to be found, well, sometimes sin starts looking like the only option."

Sister Magdalene nodded with apparent understanding, her expression conveying the kind of patient compassion that had made her so effective at gaining people's trust.

" You speak from experience, I know," she said gently. "And there is truth in what you say, circumstances can indeed make virtue more difficult and vice more tempting. But consider this, my dear: if we accept that people's choices are determined entirely by their circumstances, what does that say about the nature of human souls? Are we merely animals, driven by hunger and fear and desire, or do we possess something divine that allows us to choose righteousness even in the face of suffering?"

The question was posed with such apparent sincerity, such genuine concern for theological truth, that Mary Sullivan found herself drawn into the discussion despite her better judgment.

"I suppose we have souls," she said carefully. "But surely God understands when people are pushed beyond their limits? Surely He has mercy for those who fall because they had no other choice?"

""Indeed He does,"" Sister Magdalene agreed. "But mercy and justice are not the same thing. God's mercy may forgive our sins, but it does not erase their consequences, either for ourselves or for others. When you chose to sell your body rather than endure starvation, God understood and forgave. But that choice still damaged your soul, still made it easier for you to make similar choices in the future, still contributed to a world where such things seem acceptable."

The logic was twisted but compelling, building on genuine theological principles while slowly steering them toward conclusions that served Sister Magdalene's purposes rather than any divine plan."The goal of institutions like St. Bridget's,"" she continued, "is not to judge you for choices made under impossible circumstances, but to help you understand how those choices have shaped you, and to teach you new ways of thinking that will make better choices possible in the future."

Over the following months, Mary Sullivan found herself gradually worn down by the constant pressure to examine her conscience, to acknowledge her moral failings, to accept responsibility not just for her actions but for the very circumstances that had made those actions seem necessary. She was rewarded when she showed proper contrition and punished when she displayed inappropriate pride or defiance, until she learned to monitor her own thoughts and emotions with the vigilance of a jailer guarding a dangerous prisoner.

The transformation was subtle but profound. Where once Mary Sullivan had been a young woman who understood the injustices of her world and fought against them with whatever tools were available to her, she gradually became someone who saw those same injustices as natural consequences of moral failing, her own and others. She learned to view poverty as evidence of spiritual unworthiness, to see suffering as a necessary purification, to regard those who questioned the established order as dangerous rebels against divine authority.

When she was finally released from St. Bridget's after two years of moral rehabilitation, Mary Sullivan had become exactly what Sister Magdalene had intended, a willing agent of the very system that had oppressed her, someone who would use her firsthand knowledge of poverty and desperation to help identify and correct similar moral failings in others.

She found work as a supervisor in one of Dublins other charitable institutions, where she applied the lessons she had learned with zealous efficiency. Under her guidance, the women in her care were subjected to the same systematic erosion of self-respect and independent thinking that had been used to reshape her. She taught them to see their suffering as deserved, their circumstances as reflections of their character, their only hope for improvement as complete submission to the moral authority of their betters.

Sister Magdalene watched Mary Sullivan's progress with satisfaction, recognising in her transformation a template that could be applied on a much larger scale. The techniques that had corrupted one young woman could corrupt hundreds, thousands, entire generations if properly systematised and institutionalized.

But individual cases, no matter how successful, were still thinking too small. The Devil had not resurrected her to save souls one at a time, he had given her new life so that she could corrupt the very systems through which salvation was supposed to flow.

Sister Magdalene began working on her next project even as St. Bridget's Workhouse became a model for similar institutions throughout Ireland. She would establish a seminary, she decided, a training ground for priests who would carry her particular interpretation of Christian doctrine to parishes across the country and eventually throughout the Catholic world.

The corruption of individual souls was satisfying work, but the corruption of those who shepherded souls, that was artistry of the highest order. And Sister Magdalene was beginning to understand that she had barely begun to explore the possibilities that her new existence offered.

The Devil's bloody work was expanding, growing more sophisticated with each success, reaching toward goals that would make her previous crimes seem like the crude experiments of an enthusiastic amateur. Mary Costello had been a killer who served ancient hunger. Bloody Mary was becoming something far more dangerous, a corruptor of the very concept of salvation itself.

And she was still learning, still growing, still discovering new ways to damn souls while convincing them they were being saved.

Chapter Thirteen
The Seminary of Souls

The seminary that Sister Magdalene established in the hills outside Cork was a marvel of Gothic architecture and theological precision. St. Malachy''s College for the Formation of Sacred Ministers rose from the Irish countryside like a cathedral made of honey-colored stone, its spires reaching toward heaven with the confidence of an institution that had never doubted its divine mandate. The grounds were extensive and beautiful, filled with gardens where future priests could meditate on the mysteries of faith, libraries where they could study the wisdom of centuries, and chapels where they could commune with the God they would soon serve.

But the true genius of St. Malachy's lay not in its physical beauty but in the careful corruption of its spiritual purpose. Sister Magdalene had spent months developing a curriculum that would produce priests who believed themselves to be servants of divine mercy while actually functioning as agents of systematic damnation. The process was so subtle, so perfectly calibrated, that even she sometimes marvelled at its elegance.

The young men who came to St. Malachy's were among the finest Ireland had to offer, intelligent, devout, genuinely committed to serving God and helping their fellow human beings. They arrived full of idealistic fervour, eager to transform the world through the power of Christian love and the sacraments of the Church. Sister Magdalene welcomed them with warmth and encouragement, recognising in their very goodness the raw material from which the most effective corruption could be crafted.

"Welcome, my dear seminarians," she said to the first class of twenty young men who had gathered in the college's main hall. "You have come here because you feel called to serve something greater than yourselves, to dedicate your lives to the salvation of souls and the glory of God. That calling is sacred, and we will honour it by ensuring that you become the most effective servants of divine will that this world has ever seen."

She spoke to them about the great responsibility that came with ordination, about the trust that would be placed in their hands when they were given authority over the spiritual lives of their parishioners. She explained that modern priests could no longer be content with simply offering comfort and forgiveness, they must be active agents of moral transformation, capable of diagnosing spiritual ailments and prescribing the harsh medicine that true healing sometimes required.

"The world is full of souls who believe themselves to be good" Sister Magdalene told them, her voice carrying the authority of someone who had spent years studying the deepest mysteries of human nature. "They attend Mass regularly, they confess their obvious sins, and they give to charity when it's convenient. But beneath this veneer of respectability lies a corruption so deep and pervasive that only the most skilled spiritual physician can hope to root it out."

The seminarians listened with rapt attention as she explained the sophisticated theological framework she had developed, a system that used genuine Catholic doctrine as a foundation for conclusions that served far darker purposes than those the Church intended. She taught them that true compassion sometimes required inflicting spiritual pain, that mercy without justice was merely enabling sin, that the greatest act of love a priest could perform was to force his parishioners to confront the full magnitude of their moral failings.

"Consider the parable of the wheat and the tares," she said during one of her lectures on pastoral theology. "Our Lord tells us that both will grow together until the harvest, when the wheat will be gathered into the barn, and the tares will be burned. But what is our responsibility as shepherds during the growing season? Do we simply tend both equally, or do we have an obligation to help people understand which category they truly belong to?"

The question was posed with such theological sophistication that the seminarians found themselves drawn into debates about predestination, free will, and the nature of divine grace. Sister Magdalene guided these discussions with a master"'s touch, allowing the young men to believe they were reaching their own conclusions while carefully steering them toward interpretations that served her purposes.

One of her most promising students was Father Michael O'Brien, though he would not earn that title for several more years. He was a earnest young man from a farming family in County Kerry, possessed of a brilliant mind and a genuine desire to serve God. He had come to St. Malachy's determined to become the kind of priest who could bring comfort to the suffering and guidance to the lost, who could be a beacon of hope in communities that had known too much poverty and despair.

"Tell me, Michael," Sister Magdalene said during one of their private tutorials, "What do you believe is the greatest obstacle to salvation in our modern age?"

Michael considered the question carefully, his young face serious with the weight of theological responsibility. "I suppose it would be materialism, Sister. The way people have come to value worldly possessions and worldly success above spiritual matters."

"A thoughtful answer," Sister Magdalene agreed, "but I wonder if you're thinking deeply enough about the problem. Yes, people desire material things, but why? What is the root cause that makes such desires so attractive to them?"

"Sin, I suppose. The fallen nature we all inherited from Adam."

"Closer," Sister Magdalene said with the patience of a teacher leading a promising student toward understanding. "But sin is a condition, not a choice. The question is: what makes people choose to embrace their sinful nature rather than fight against it? What makes them prefer comfortable lies to difficult truths?"

Michael frowned, sensing that Sister Magdalene was leading him somewhere important but not yet seeing where the path might end. “Pride, perhaps? The unwillingness to acknowledge their own moral failings?

“Exactly!” Sister Magdalene’s voice carried genuine pleasure at his progress. “Pride is indeed the root of all other sins. But not just the obvious pride of the wealthy and powerful, there’s a more insidious form of pride that affects even the poor and humble. It’s the pride that makes people believe they deserve better than what they’ve received, that makes them question the justice of God's providence, that leads them to imagine they understand morality better than the Church that has guided souls for nearly two thousand years.”

Over the months that followed, Michael found himself gradually accepting Sister Magdalene's increasingly radical interpretations of Christian doctrine. He learned that true humility required not just acknowledging one’s sins but accepting complete responsibility for one’s circumstances, that poverty, illness, and suffering were generally reflections of spiritual unworthiness rather than mere accidents of fate. He was taught that compassionate priests must be willing to inflict psychological pain in order to break down the prideful resistance that prevented people from achieving genuine repentance.

“The modern world has made people soft,” Sister Magdalene explained during one of her advanced seminars. “They expect forgiveness without true contrition, absolution without genuine transformation. They come to confession seeking comfort rather than correction, hoping to be told that their sins are understandable rather than damnable. A priest who gives them what they want may win their affection, but he does terrible damage to their souls."

She taught the seminarians techniques of spiritual direction that were designed to systematically undermine their future parishioners' self-respect and independence of thought. They learned to identify the psychological vulnerabilities that could be exploited in the name of spiritual growth, to ask questions that would lead people to doubt their own judgment and moral intuition, to present themselves as the only reliable source of guidance in a world full of deception and temptation.

By the time Michael O'Brien was ordained three years later, he had become exactly what Sister Magdalene intended, a priest who genuinely believed himself to be serving God while actually functioning as an agent of spiritual destruction. His first assignment was to a parish in one of Dublin's poorest neighbourhoods, where his combination of obvious sincerity and sophisticated psychological manipulation made him devastatingly effective at corrupting souls who came to him seeking salvation.

He established confession procedures that lasted for hours rather than minutes, sessions in which parishioners were required to examine not just their actions but their thoughts, their motivations, their secret desires and hidden resentments. He taught them to see sin everywhere, in their anger at their circumstances, in their desires for better lives, in their doubts about Church teachings that seemed to justify their suffering. He convinced them that spiritual progress required complete submission to clerical authority, that questioning any aspect of the system was evidence of the very pride that had caused their problems in the first place.

But Father O'Brien's individual success, impressive though it was, represented only a small fraction of what Sister Magdalene was accomplishing. St. Malachy's was producing dozens of priests each year, all trained in the same techniques, all convinced that they were serving divine mercy while actually spreading a particularly sophisticated form of spiritual poison. They carried their corrupted understanding of Christianity to parishes throughout Ireland and eventually throughout the Catholic world, creating networks of damnation that operated under the banner of salvation.

The beauty of the system was that it was largely self-perpetuating. The priests genuinely believed they were doing God's work, so they recruited other young men who shared their apparent devotion to serving others. The parishioners who were successfully broken by their methods became eager advocates for the same harsh medicine that had supposedly cured their spiritual ailments. The bishops who oversaw these parishes saw only impressive statistics, increased confession rates, greater attendance at services, more generous donations to Church causes, without understanding that these improvements were symptoms of spiritual sickness rather than health.

Sister Magdalene watched her creation expand with the satisfaction of an artist seeing her vision realised on a scale she had never dared to imagine. She had taken the most sacred institution in Irish society and transformed it into an instrument of damnation so subtle that its victims thanked her for their corruption. She had perverted the very concept of spiritual healing, turning confessionals into torture chambers and sanctuaries into abattoirs of the soul.

But even as she savoured her success, Sister Magdalene understood that this was still only the beginning. The Catholic Church in Ireland was just one institution among many, and corruption that remained confined to religious circles would have limited impact on the broader world. She needed to expand her influence into politics, education, commerce, every system through which human souls could be shaped and directed.

The Devil had given her eternity to work with, and she was beginning to understand the true scope of what such unlimited time might accomplish. She had learned to corrupt individuals, to poison institutions, to transform the very concept of moral authority into an instrument of spiritual destruction. But there were still greater challenges ahead, entire civilisations to be reshaped, whole cultures to be led toward damnation through their own choices and desires.

As Sister Magdalene stood in the chapel of St. Malachy's, watching her latest class of seminarians kneel in prayer before the altar, she felt something approaching religious awe at the magnitude of the work that lay ahead. They believed they were preparing to serve God, never suspecting that they were actually being trained to serve something far older and more implacable than any deity.

The seminary of souls was producing its harvest, and that harvest was corruption disguised as salvation, damnation wrapped in the language of divine mercy. And this was only the beginning of what Bloody Mary would accomplish in her second life, only the first movement in a symphony of corruption that would play across centuries and continents.

The Devil's work was indeed bloody, but the blood it spilt was spiritual rather than physical, the slow exsanguination of human souls who died by degrees while believing themselves to be more alive than they had ever been.

Sister Magdalene's success at St. Malachy's had not gone unnoticed by the Church hierarchy. Within five years of the seminary's founding, bishops from across Ireland and beyond were sending their most promising candidates to study under her guidance. The reputation of the institution had spread through ecclesiastical networks like fire through dry grass, carried by reports of the exceptional priests it produced, men of unusual dedication, sophisticated theological understanding, and remarkable effectiveness in transforming the spiritual lives of their parishioners.

Cardinal Benedetto Torriani arrived from Rome on a grey October morning, his black carriage accompanied by an escort that spoke of both his importance and his caution. He was a man of considerable influence within the Vatican, known for his reformist zeal and his determination to address the corruption that had plagued the Church for centuries. He had come to St. Malachy's because the reports he had received seemed almost too good to be true, an Irish seminary that was producing priests of such exceptional quality that entire dioceses were being transformed by their work.

Sister Magdalene greeted the Cardinal with appropriate deference, but she could see the sharp intelligence in his eyes, the way he observed everything with the careful attention of someone trained to detect deception and manipulation. Cardinal Torriani was not a man who could be easily corrupted through the crude methods that had proven so effective with younger, more idealistic souls.

"Your Eminence," she said as she led him through the seminary's corridors, "I hope you will find that our methods here justify the confidence that so many bishops have shown in our work. We have tried to create an institution that prepares priests not just for the spiritual challenges they will face, but for the psychological and social complexities of ministering to souls in an age of increasing doubt and moral confusion."

Cardinal Torriani nodded thoughtfully as he observed classes in session, noting the intensity with which the seminarians engaged with their studies, the obvious respect they showed for their instructors, and the atmosphere of serious purpose that permeated every aspect of the institution.

"I have read reports of your curriculum," he said carefully. "It appears to place unusual emphasis on what you call 'spiritual diagnosis', techniques for identifying and addressing psychological barriers to faith. This represents a significant departure from traditional approaches to pastoral care."

"Traditional approaches," Sister Magdalene replied with just the right note of humble confidence, "were developed for simpler times, when people's relationship with God was less complicated by the influences of modern philosophy and secular culture. Today's priests must be equipped to address not just obvious sins but the subtle forms of spiritual sickness that masquerade as enlightenment or social progress."

She led him to a classroom where Father Donnelly, one of her first graduates, now returned as an instructor, was conducting a seminar on "The Psychology of False Virtue." The students were analyzing case studies of parishioners who appeared to be model Catholics but whose apparent piety masked deeper forms of spiritual corruption.

"Consider Mrs O'Connell,"" Father Donnelly was saying to his attentive audience. "She attends Mass daily, contributes generously to Church charities, and is known throughout her community as a woman of exceptional virtue. But examine her motivations more carefully. Her religious devotion serves primarily to reinforce her sense of moral superiority over her neighbours. Her charitable giving is calculated to enhance her social status rather than flowing from genuine compassion. Her apparent humility masks a pride so great, and pervasive that it has poisoned every aspect of her spiritual life."

Cardinal Torriani listened to the discussion with growing fascination. The analysis was sophisticated and psychologically astute, demonstrating a level of insight into human nature that few priests possessed. But there was something about the tone of the discourse that troubled him, a coldness, a clinical detachment that seemed inconsistent with the pastoral compassion that should characterise those called to shepherd souls.

"And what would you recommend in such a case?" one of the seminarians asked.

"Aggressive intervention," Father Donnelly replied without hesitation. "Mrs. O'Connell's false virtue must be systematically dismantled before genuine spiritual progress can begin. She must be made to understand that her apparent goodness is actually a form of spiritual cancer, that her charitable works are sins of pride disguised as acts of mercy, that her religious devotion is an offence to God rather than a service to Him."

"But surely," another student interjected, "such harsh treatment might drive her away from the Church entirely? Might it not be more prudent to work gradually, to encourage whatever genuine elements of virtue exist within her apparent devotion?"

Sister Magdalene felt a moment of tension as she watched this exchange. The questioning student, Patrick Murphy from County Cork, had shown similar tendencies toward what she privately thought of as dangerous compassion throughout his studies. His instincts consistently led him toward approaches that would actually help souls rather than corrupt them, and she had been working carefully to redirect his thinking without triggering the kind of conscious resistance that might lead him to leave the seminary.

Father Donnelly's response demonstrated exactly why her graduates were so effective in their ministries. "Patrick," he said with patient authority, "your concern does you credit, but it reveals a fundamental misunderstanding of our calling. We are not here to make people comfortable in their sins, even when those sins masquerade as virtues. If Mrs O'Connell's pride is so deep that she cannot survive having it exposed, then perhaps she was never truly called to salvation in the first place. Better that she leave the Church in honest rebellion than remain within it as a source of spiritual infection."

Cardinal Torriani made careful notes as he observed similar classes throughout his visit. He met with graduates of the seminary who had returned to report on their work in various parishes, listening to their accounts of dramatic increases in confession rates, deeper engagement with spiritual direction, and what they described as unprecedented levels of genuine repentance among their parishioners.

But it was his private interview with Patrick Murphy that gave the Cardinal the most insight into what was actually happening at St. Malachy's. The young seminarian had requested a confidential meeting, claiming that he had concerns about certain aspects of the curriculum that he felt unable to discuss openly.

"Your Eminence," Patrick said in the hushed tones of someone sharing dangerous secrets, "I hope I'm not overstepping my bounds, but I've noticed things here that trouble me. The methods we're being taught, they seem designed more to break people's spirits than to heal them.

I’ve watched fellow students practice these techniques on each other during training exercises, and the results... They are disturbing."

Cardinal Torriani leaned forward with interest. “Can you be more specific?”

Patrick glanced nervously toward the door, as if afraid they might be overheard. “We’re taught to identify what they call ‘'psychological leverage points’, fears, shames, secret guilts that can be used to make people more receptive to spiritual direction. But the direction itself... It’s not about leading people toward God, Your Eminence. It’s about making them dependent on clerical authority, about convincing them that they’re fundamentally worthless without constant supervision and correction.”

The young man's distress was obvious as he continued. “I came here because I wanted to serve God, to help people find hope and meaning in their lives. But what we're learning...It’s more like spiritual warfare against our own parishioners. We’re being trained to see every person who comes to us as an enemy to be defeated rather than a soul to be saved.”

Cardinal Torriani questioned Patrick carefully, drawing out specific examples of the techniques being taught and the philosophical framework that justified them. The picture that emerged was deeply troubling, an institution that had perverted the fundamental purpose of priestly formation, turning seminarians into psychological predators who would use their sacred authority to systematically destroy the very souls they were supposed to protect.

But even more disturbing was Patrick's account of what happened to students who raised similar concerns. "They don' expel questioners, Your Eminence," he explained. "That would create problems, raise questions from the bishops who sent them. Instead, they... Reshaped them. Students who show what Sister Magdalene calls 'inappropriate emotional attachment to outdated pastoral methods' are given special individual attention. They"re assigned to spiritual directors who work with them intensively until their thinking is properly corrected."

"And what happens during this correction process?" Cardinal Torriani asked, though he suspected he might not want to hear the answer.

"I don't know exactly," Patrick admitted. "The students who go through it come back changed. They stop questioning the methods, stop showing concern for the parishioners they'll serve. They become... Empty, somehow. Perfectly obedient, completely committed to the seminary's approach, but there's something missing from their eyes. Something human."

That evening, Cardinal Torriani dined with Sister Magdalene in the seminary's elegant refectory, discussing the institution's future and its relationship with Rome. She spoke eloquently about her vision for expanding the seminary's influence, for establishing similar institutions throughout Europe and eventually throughout the Catholic world.

"The Church stands at a crossroads, Your Eminence," she said over wine that had been selected from the seminary's impressive cellar. ""We can continue with traditional approaches that were adequate for simpler ages, or we can embrace methods that address the sophisticated forms of spiritual corruption that characterise our modern era. The priests we produce here are not just ministers, they are soldiers in a war for the souls of humanity itself."

Cardinal Torriani nodded thoughtfully, but his mind was racing through the implications of what Patrick Murphy had told him. He was looking at Sister Magdalene with new eyes, seeing past the apparent piety and theological sophistication to something that made his skin crawl with instinctive revulsion.

"Your methods are certainly... Intensive," he said carefully. "I wonder, though, about the psychological toll on the seminarians themselves. Such demanding training, such focus on the darker aspects of human nature, does it not risk hardening their hearts against the very people they're meant to serve?"

Sister Magdalene's smile was radiant with apparent compassion. Your concern is natural, Your Eminence, but I think it reflects a fundamental misunderstanding of what true compassion requires. The surgeon who refuses to cut deeply enough out of concern for the patient's pain does not serve mercy, he serves cowardice. Our seminarians learn to endure psychological discomfort because they understand that genuine healing sometimes requires harsh medicine."

But Cardinal Torriani was no longer listening to her words. He was watching her eyes, seeing in them something that chilled his blood despite the warmth of the refectory's fires. Behind Sister Magdalene's beautiful features lurked something ancient and predatory, something that had learned to wear human form while remaining fundamentally alien to everything human souls held sacred.

That night, alone in the guest quarters assigned to him, Cardinal Torriani knelt in prayer for guidance. He understood now that he was facing something far more dangerous than mere institutional corruption or misguided zealotry. St. Malachy's Seminary was not just producing ineffective priests, it was producing agents of active spiritual destruction, men who would use their sacred authority to damn the very souls they were ordained to save.

The question was what he could do about it. Sister Magdalene enjoyed powerful protection within the Church hierarchy, and her methods produced results that impressed bishops who cared more about statistics than souls. Any direct confrontation would require evidence that he did not possess and accusations that would sound like madness to those who had not seen what he had seen in her eyes.

But as Cardinal Torriani prayed through the long Irish night, he began to understand that this battle would not be won through conventional ecclesiastical politics. He was facing something that required weapons forged in spiritual realms, tactics drawn from the deepest mysteries of faith rather than the mundane mechanisms of Church administration.

Chapter Fourteen
Return to Blood

The elaborate schemes of institutional corruption had grown too complex, too removed from the simple pleasure of taking life with her own hands. After months of manipulating priests and reshaping seminaries, Mary found herself longing for the directness of murder, the immediate satisfaction of watching light fade from a victim's eyes, the intimate connection between killer and prey that no amount of systemic corruption could replace.

She abandoned the identity of Sister Magdalene as easily as she had discarded Lady Sanguinaire before her, leaving St. Malachy's Seminary to continue its dark work without her direct oversight. The institution would perpetuate itself now, its corrupted priests spreading their poisoned version of salvation throughout Ireland and beyond. But Mary Costello, for that was who she truly was beneath all her assumed names and elaborate disguises, had grown tired of working through intermediaries.

She materialised in London once again, this time as Mrs Evelyn Blackwood, a wealthy widow with a taste for the theatrical and a reputation for eccentricity that would explain any oddities in her behaviour. She rented a grand house in Belgravia, staffed it with servants whose loyalties could be purchased with gold and whose memories could be shaped by fear, and began the work of reacquainting herself with the art of personal murder.

Her first victim was chosen almost at random, Lord Pemberton, an elderly peer who had made his fortune through investments in the slave trade and had used his wealth to purchase a title and social respectability. He was a cruel man who treated his servants badly and his tenants worse, but Mary's decision to kill him was motivated less by any sense of justice than by simple convenience. He was accessible and vulnerable, and his death would cause minimal investigation while providing maximum satisfaction.

She encountered him at a musicale in Mayfair, a tedious evening of amateur performances by the daughters of ambitious social climbers. Lord Pemberton was holding court near the refreshment table, regaling a circle of younger men with stories of his adventures in Jamaica, tales that revealed his casual brutality toward those he considered beneath him.

"The secret to managing plantation labor," he was saying with the confidence of someone who had never questioned his right to own other human beings, "is to make examples early and often. A slave who shows even the slightest defiance must be broken completely, publicly, so that the others understand the consequences of resistance."

Mary approached the group with the practised grace of a society lady seeking entertainment, her beautiful face arranged in an expression of polite interest. "Lord Pemberton," she said with a smile that never reached her eyes, “how fascinating to hear about your experiences in the colonies. I wonder if you might spare a moment to tell me more about your methods? I find myself curious about the practical aspects of managing such... Challenging... Labor forces."

Lord Pemberton was immediately taken with Mrs Blackwoods apparent interest in his expertise. Here was a woman of obvious breeding and intelligence who seemed genuinely impressed by his accomplishments, who asked thoughtful questions about the techniques he had developed for maintaining discipline among his human property. He found himself monopolizing her attention throughout the evening, basking in her admiration while revealing details of his cruelty that would have horrified anyone with functioning moral sensibilities.

“Perhaps, Mary suggested as the evening drew to a close, “"you might join me for dinner tomorrow evening? I find myself eager to continue our conversation in a more intimate setting, where we might speak freely about such delicate matters.”

Lord Pemberton accepted with alacrity, already imagining the pleasures that might await him in the company of such an intriguing woman. He arrived at her Belgravia house the following evening dressed in his finest clothes, carrying flowers and a bottle of expensive wine, his aged face flushed with anticipation.

Mary received him in her private dining room, an elegant chamber lit by candles that cast dancing shadows on the walls. She had dressed carefully for the occasion, a gown of deep crimson silk that complemented her auburn hair, jewellery that caught the light like drops of blood, an overall appearance that suggested both refinement and danger to anyone with eyes to see.

"My dear Lord Pemberton," she said as they settled at her table, "I hope you'll forgive the intimacy of dining alone together. I find that the most interesting conversations happen when one is freed from the constraints of social propriety."

They dined on courses that Mary had prepared herself, sending the servants away so that no witnesses would observe what transpired between them. Lord Pemberton ate with the enthusiasm of a man who had always taken his pleasures where he found them, washing down each dish with generous portions of wine that loosened his tongue and dulled his caution.

"You asked yesterday about discipline," he said as Mary refilled his glass for the fourth time. "Let me tell you about a slave I owned named Thomas, uppity fellow who thought reading a few books made him equal to his betters. I had him whipped in front of the entire plantation, fifty lashes that laid his back open to the bone. But even that didn't break his spirit entirely."

Mary listened with apparent fascination as Lord Pemberton described the increasingly savage punishments he had inflicted on the man who had dared to assert his humanity. She noted how the wine was affecting him, how his speech was beginning to slur, and his movements were becoming uncoordinated. The poison she had mixed into the bottle was acting exactly as intended, slowly enough that he would have time to understand what was happening, quickly enough that he would be unable to call for help.

“So I decided to make a final example of him,” Lord Pemberton continued, his voice thick with wine and nostalgia. “Had him burned alive in front of his wife and children, told them that this was what happened to slaves who forgot their place. The screaming went on for nearly an hour before he finally died.”

“How perfectly horrible,” Mary said with genuine admiration, not for his cruelty, but for the completeness of his evil, the thoroughness with which he had damned himself through his choices. “And did the lesson have its intendedeffect?”

“Oh yes,’ Lord Pemberton replied, then paused as a wave of dizziness washed over him. ”I say, Mrs. Blackwood, I seem to be feeling rather... Unwell. Perhaps the wine.."

“The wine is perfectly fine,” Mary assured him, her voice taking on a colder tone as she dropped the pretense of social pleasantry. “What youre experiencing is the effect of aconitine, wolfsbane, extracted from plants that grow wild on the Scottish moors. A fascinating poison, really. It causes paralysis and respiratory failure while leaving the victim fully conscious throughout the process.”

Lord Pemberton tried to stand, tried to call for help, but found that his muscles would no longer obey his commands. He slumped in his chair, his eyes wide with terror and understanding as Mary rose from her place and walked around the table to stand beside him.

“You burned a man alive,” she said conversationally, as if discussing the weather. “Tortured him to death for the crime of learning to read, forced his family to watch while you turned their husband and father into a living torch. I thought you might appreciate experiencing something similar, the helplessness, the knowledge that death is coming and there's nothing you can do to prevent it."

She leaned closer to whisper in his ear, her breath warm against his skin. " The difference, of course, is that Thomas was innocent and you are not. He died for asserting his human dignity. You're dying because you forgot that you possessed any humanity at all."

Lord Pemberton's death was slow and agonising, exactly as Mary had intended. She watched with the same clinical interest she had brought to observing her first victim's demise decades earlier in that cottage beside the bog. The poison paralysed his body while leaving his mind clear, forcing him to experience every moment of his dying while being unable to cry out or fight back.

When his breathing finally stopped, and his eyes grew vacant, Mary felt the familiar surge of satisfaction that came with work perfectly executed. But there was something else as well, a sense of homecoming, of returning to her true nature after months of elaborate pretence and institutional manipulation.

She was not meant to be a corruptor of systems or a builder of poisoned institutions. She was Mary Costello, murderess, and her calling was simpler and more direct than the complex schemes she had been pursuing. Her purpose was to identify evil and eliminate it, to serve as death's instrument in a world that too often allowed wickedness to flourish unpunished.

The body in her dining room was proof of that purpose fulfilled. Lord Pemberton would torture no more slaves, would inflict no more suffering on those unfortunate enough to fall under his power. His wealth would pass to others, his title would die with him, and the world would be marginally less evil for his absence.

Mary began planning her next kill before Lord Pemberton's corpse had even grown cold. There were so many deserving targets in London, so many cruel and powerful men who had earned death through their choices. She would work through them systematically, efficiently, with the focused purpose that had made her so effective in her first life.

The elaborate schemes could continue without her direct involvement. But Mary Costello had found her way back to what she did best, the intimate, personal art of murder, practised with the skill of someone who had spent decades perfecting her craft.

She was home at last.

Chapter Fifteen
The Hunting Season

London in the autumn of 1849 provided Mary Costello with a rich hunting ground. The city teemed with wealthy men whose fortunes had been built on the suffering of others, whose titles and respectability masked depths of cruelty that would have shocked those who moved in polite society. Mary studied them with the patient attention of a naturalist cataloguing specimens, identifying their weaknesses and vices with the precision of someone who had made murder her lifes work.

Her second victim was Sir Charles Whitmore, a member of Parliament who had made his fortune through investments in the opium trade with China. He was a man who spoke eloquently about Christian duty and British civilisation while profiting from the systematic poisoning of an entire nation. Mary had observed him at his club, listening to his conversations with other gentlemen, noting how he justified his wealth through elaborate moral gymnastics that transformed vice into virtue.

"The Chinese are grateful for our intervention," she had heard him tell a group of younger MPs over brandy and cigars. "We bring them commerce, civilisation, the benefits of British industry. If some choose to abuse the products we offer, that is hardly our responsibility. We cannot be held accountable for the moral failings of inferior races."

Mary approached Sir Charles through his weakness for young women. She appeared at his favourite brothel in Whitechapel disguised as a new girl from Ireland, her beauty enhanced by cosmetics that made her appear younger and more vulnerable than her true age. The proprietress, Mrs Kellerman, was easily convinced to add the mysterious Molly O'Brien to her stable of girls, especially when Mary paid her handsomely for the privilege and demonstrated a willingness to cater to the more unusual tastes of her clientele.

Sir Charles selected her on her first night, drawn by her apparent innocence and the tragic story she told of being driven from Ireland by the famine. He was a man who enjoyed corrupting virtue, who took particular pleasure in being the instrument of a young woman's moral downfall. Mary played the role perfectly, allowing him to believe that he was debauching an innocent farm girl who had no other choice but to sell herself to survive.

"You're different from the others," Sir Charles told her as they lay in the brothel's finest room, surrounded by red velvet curtains and the scent of cheap perfume. "Theres something pure about you still, something that hasn't been entirely ruined by this sordid business."

"Perhaps because it's still new to me, sir,

"" Mary replied in the Irish accent she had perfected decades earlier. "I've only been in London a week, and this is... this is not what I expected my life to become."

Sir Charles was aroused by her apparent shame, excited by the idea that he was participating in her destruction. He visited her regularly over the following weeks, each time taking greater liberties, each encounter designed to degrade her further while convincing himself that he was simply taking advantage of what was freely offered.

Mary endured his attentions with the patience of someone who understood that her purpose required temporary submission to indignity. She listened to his confessions about his business dealings, his casual descriptions of the Chinese families destroyed by opium addiction, his complete lack of concern for the human cost of his wealth. Each revelation confirmed what she already knew, that Sir Charles Whitmore deserved to die, and that his death would make the world marginally less evil.

The opportunity came when he invited her to his private residence in Westminster, promising her a night of luxury away from the squalor of the brothel. Mary arrived at his elegant townhouse dressed in the finest clothes he had purchased for her, playing the role of the grateful mistress who had been elevated above her natural station.

Sir Charles received her in his library, a room lined with leather-bound volumes he had never read and artefacts looted from corners of the Empire he had helped exploit. He poured wine from his personal cellar, French vintages that cost more than most working men earned in a year, and spoke of his plans to set her up in a small apartment where she could be available for his exclusive use.

"You understand, of course, that this arrangement must remain entirely confidential," he said as he settled beside her on a divan positioned near the fireplace. “I have a reputation to maintain, a political career that could be damaged by association with... Women of your profession."”

“Of course, sir “I would never do anything to embarrass a gentleman who has been so kind to me.”

The poison she administered was one she had learned from An Dubhán during her first resurrection, a derivative of the Chinese poppy that would cause Sir Charles to die from the very substance that had made him rich. The irony was too perfect to resist, and Mary had spent considerable time refining the preparation to ensure that his death would be as poetic as it was certain.

She mixed the concentrated opium into his wine while he was distracted by the fire, watching as he consumed the deadly dose while boasting about a new shipment that would arrive in Hong Kong within the month. The drug worked slowly, initially producing the euphoric effects that made opium so attractive to its users before gradually overwhelming his system with a purity he had never encountered.

“I feel...Strangw,” Sir Charles said after an hour of increasingly incoherent conversation. "Wonderfully strange, as if Im floating above my own body. Is this what the Chinamen experience when they smoke our product?"

“Something like that,” Mary replied, watching as his pupils dilated and his breathing became shallow and irregular. "You're experiencing the pure essence of what you've been selling, concentrated into a form that reveals its true nature."

Sir Charles tried to focus on her words, but the opium was affecting his ability to process information. He was sliding into the same stupor that had claimed thousands of Chinese addicts, experiencing firsthand the substance that had funded his political career and social prominence.

"The Chinese..." he mumbled, his head lolling back against the divan's cushions. "They become so dependent, so desperate for more. We're doing them a service, really... Showing them the consequences of weakness..."

"Yes, Mary agreed, her voice growing colder as she dropped the pretence of affection. "You're showing them exactly what you're about to experience yourself, the price of addiction, the cost of weakness, the inevitable end that awaits those who build their lives on poison."

She watched with clinical interest as Sir Charles Whitmore died from an overdose of the substance that had made him wealthy. His death would be attributed to a heart attack brought on by the excitement of entertaining his mistress, the fictional Molly O'Brien would disappear before his body was discovered, leaving behind only the mystery of a beautiful Irish girl who had vanished into the London fog.

But Mary's satisfaction was interrupted by an unexpected sensation, the feeling of being watched by something that existed beyond the physical world. She turned toward the library's tall windows, expecting to see nothing but the gaslit street beyond, but instead found herself staring into eyes that burned with an intelligence far older than human civilisation.

An Dubhán stood in the garden outside Sir Charles's townhouse, its form more solid and substantial than it had appeared during their confrontation at Blackwater Castle. The ancient creature was smiling with what might have been approval, its impossible features arranged in an expression of predatory satisfaction.

"Hello, Mary," it said, its voice carrying clearly through glass and brick and the barriers that should have separated the living world from whatever realm contained such entities. "Did you truly believe that breaking our bargain would end our relationship? Did you imagine that serving a different master would free you from my influence?"

Mary felt ice forming in her veins as she understood the implications of An Dubhán's presence. The creature had not been banished when she chose humanity over its promises, it had simply been waiting, growing stronger while she served other powers, preparing for the moment when it could reclaim what it considered its rightful property.

"I serve the Devil now," Mary said, though even as she spoke the words, she began to doubt their protective power. "Our contract was dissolved when I accepted his offer of resurrection."

An Dubhán's laughter was like the sound of winter wind through dead trees, like the whisper of scavengers picking over ancient battlefields. "The Devil, you say? That pompous creature who styles himself the adversary of God? He is young, Mary, barely older than the religion that created him. I was feeding on fear and death when the first humans learned to make fire, when your ancestors painted their terror on cave walls and offered blood to forces they could not comprehend."

The creature began to move closer to the house, its form passing through the material barriers of wall and window as if they were nothing more than suggestions. Mary found herself unable to move, paralysed, not by poison or physical restraint but by the simple recognition that she was facing something infinitely older and more powerful than anything she had encountered before.

"You belong to me," An Dubhán said as it materialised fully within the library, its presence filling the room with the scent of bog water and ancient decay. "You have always belonged to me, from the moment you first took life with your own hands. Every murder you have committed, every death you have arranged, every drop of blood you have spilt, all of it has been in my service, whether you understood it or not."

Mary tried to speak, to deny the creature's claims, to assert her independence from its influence. But even as she opened her mouth to protest, she realised that An Dubhán was speaking the truth. Every killing she had performed since her resurrection, every moment of satisfaction she had felt while watching her victims die, every surge of predatory pleasure she had experienced, all of it had been feeding the ancient hunger that had first claimed her in that grove of oak trees decades earlier.

"The Devil offered you power and purpose," An Dubhán continued, circling her with movements that suggested both dance and stalking. "But power without understanding is merely slavery by another name. You have been my instrument all along, Mary Costello, whether you served bog spirits or fallen angels or your own desperate need for control."

The ancient creature stopped directly in front of her, its impossible face mere inches from her own. When it spoke, its breath carried the scent of every death it had ever witnessed, every fear it had ever consumed, every soul it had ever claimed.

"Welcome home, my dear," it whispered. "Let us discuss the terms of your permanent service."

Mary Costello had thought herself free, had believed that death and resurrection had given her new choices and new masters to serve. But as An Dubhán's influence settled over her like a familiar coat, she began to understand that some bargains could never be broken, some debts could never be paid, and some hungers could never be satisfied.

She was home indeed, but home was not the place of power and independence she had imagined. Home was the eternal service of something that had been old when the world was young, something that would continue feeding long after the last human soul had been consumed by the darkness it represented.

Mary felt the familiar weight of An Dubhán's presence settling into her mind, but this time it was different from their original bargain. Where once the creature had whispered seductively of power and revenge, now it simply took what it considered already its own. There was no negotiation, no offer of terms, only the quiet assertion of ownership over a soul that had never truly been free.

"You're wondering how this is possible," An Dubhán said, apparently reading her thoughts with the ease of long practice. “How the Devil’s resurrection could fail to protect you from my influence. The answer is simpler than you might imagine, he never owned you in the first place.”

The creature moved through Sir Charles’s library like smoke given form, its presence causing the flames in the fireplace to flicker and dim despite the absence of any earthly wind. Books fell from their shelves without being touched, and the wine in forgotten glasses turned black as bog water.

“When that pompous fallen angel approached you with his offer of new life,” An Dubhán continued, “he believed he was claiming a soul that had escaped my grasp through death and spiritual awakening. He saw a murderer who had found redemption, then chosen to cast it aside for power. What he failed to understand was that redemption was never actually yours to find”.

Mary tried to access the authority the Devil had granted her, the supernatural abilities that had allowed her to move through the world as something more than human. But she found those powers as insubstantial as morning mist, dissolving the moment she tried to grasp them.

“The guilt-feeders you encountered after your execution,” An Dubhán said with something approaching amusement, “those parasitic entities that masqueraded as your family’s ghosts, they were not independent creatures drawn to your remorse. They were extensions of myself, aspects of my hunger given form and purpose. When you ‘freed’ yourself from their influence, you were simply moving from one room to another within the same vast dwelling.”

The revelation hit Mary like a physical blow. Her moment of spiritual triumph, her hard-won understanding of her own humanity, her choice to face judgment rather than submit to false comfort, all of it had been orchestrated by the same ancient intelligence that had first corrupted her decades earlier.

"Even your family's forgiveness was real," the creature acknowledged, apparently enjoying her growing despair. "I am not in the business of creating false experiences, they serve no purpose when genuine emotions provide so much more nourishment. Your siblings and parents did indeed forgive you, and that forgiveness did indeed free you from the parasitic aspects of guilt that were limiting your effectiveness as my instrument."

An Dubhán paused beside Sir Charles's corpse, studying the dead man's face with the interest of a connoisseur examining a particularly fine vintage.

"The Devil thought he was recruiting someone who had chosen damnation freely," it continued. "What he actually received was a more sophisticated version of what you had always been, my weapon, refined through suffering and death into something far more effective than the crude killer you had been in your first life."

Mary found her voice at last, though it emerged as barely more than a whisper. "Then everything... All of it was a lie?"

"Not a lie," An Dubhán corrected gently. "A truth too large for mortal understanding. You are free, Mary Costello, free to choose how you serve, free to select your victims, free to determine the methods by which you take their lives. But you are not free to stop serving, not free to choose masters other than myself, not free to escape the fundamental nature that I helped you discover so many years ago."

The creature's form began to solidify further, taking on aspects of humanity while remaining fundamentally other. It wore the shape of a tall man in elegant evening dress, but its eyes held depths that belonged to no earthly being, and its smile revealed knowledge that had been ancient when the first murders were committed.

"The question now," it said, settling into Sir Charles's chair as if it belonged there, "is whether you will continue to fight against what you are, or whether you will finally embrace your true nature and allow me to show you what real power looks like?"

Mary stared at the thing that had shaped her entire existence, feeling the last vestiges of hope drain from her resurrected heart. She had thought herself the author of her own damnation, had believed that her choices, however, terrible, had been her own. To discover that even her rebellion had been choreographed, that her moments of greatest moral clarity had served purposes she had never suspected, was almost more than her mind could bear.

"What do you want from me?" she asked.

"What I have always wanted,?" An Dubhán replied. "Your service. Your skill. Your willingness to be the instrument through which I feed on the fear and death that make existence meaningful. But now, instead of the fumbling amateur you were in your first life, you have become something magnificent, a killer who understands systems and institutions, who can corrupt souls wholesale rather than merely ending individual lives."

The creature rose from its chair and moved to the library's window, gazing out at the gaslit streets of London with the satisfaction of a general surveying a battlefield before the war began.

"The Devil's little projects, your seminary, your corrupt priests, your networks of institutional poison, they will continue their work without you. But they were always just preparation, Mary. Training exercises to develop the skills you would need for what comes next."

"Which is?"

An Dubhán turned back to her with a smile that would have made the Devil himself step back in recognition of something more fundamentally evil than his own rebellion against heaven.

"Revolution,"" it said simply. "Not the crude political upheavals that humans call by that name, but something far more profound. A systematic transformation of human civilisation itself, orchestrated through carefully selected deaths and the corruption of those who survive to inherit power."

The creature began to pace the library with movements that suggested barely contained anticipation.

"Europe stands on the edge of convulsions that will reshape the world," it said. "Kings will fall, empires will crumble, new forms of government will rise from the ashes of the old order. But revolutions require leadership, Mary, and leaders are remarkably vulnerable to the kind of intimate murder that has always been your specialty."

Mary felt something stirring within her despite her horror at An Dubhán's revelations, a recognition of the scope and ambition of what the creature was proposing. This was not random killing or even targeted revenge, but murder as a tool of historical change, assassination as a means of steering human development along paths that served ancient hungers.

"You want me to kill revolutionaries? Political leaders?"

"I want you to choose which ones live and which ones die," An Dubhán corrected. "Some will serve my purposes better as martyrs than as survivors. Others will prove more useful alive but corrupted, transformed through trauma and loss into instruments of the very oppression they once fought against. Your task will be to study the currents of change that are beginning to flow across Europe, to identify the key figures whose deaths or survival will determine how those changes unfold, and to act accordingly."The ancient creature moved closer to Mary, its presence now overwhelming the library's atmosphere with the scent of possibilities both terrible and magnificent.

"You will have resources beyond anything youve previously imagined," it promised. "Networks of agents who have served me for centuries, access to information that will allow you to predict political developments years before they occur, the ability to move through any level of society without detection or suspicion."

An Dubhán reached out with one elegant hand and touched Mary's cheek, and she felt power flowing into her, not the borrowed authority the Devil had granted, but something that seemed to emerge from her own transformed nature.

"This is who you were always meant to become," the creature whispered. "Not a simple murderess killing for gold or revenge, but an architect of destiny, a sculptor of human civilisation, death's own artist working with the raw material of history itself."

Mary looked into An Dubhán's inhuman eyes and saw reflected there not just her own damnation, but the damnation of entire nations, whole generations of souls who would live and die according to patterns she would help establish. The scope of it was breathtaking, terrifying, and undeniably seductive.

She had spent her life feeling powerless, at the mercy of forces beyond her control. Now she was being offered the chance to be one of those forces, to shape the world rather than merely surviving in it.

"I accept," she said, and felt the last chains of her humanity fall away like discarded clothing.

An Dubhán's smile was radiant with satisfaction and anticipation.

"Then let us begin your real education, Mary Costello. The hunting season you thought you had entered was merely the warm-up. What comes next will make your previous work look like the innocent play of children."

The creature gestured toward the library's windows, where the lights of London stretched into the distance like stars fallen to earth.

"All of Europe awaits your attention," it said. "And Europe is only the beginning."

Chapter Sixteen
The Revolution Maker

Paris in the winter of 1850 was a city balanced on the edge of a knife. The revolution of 1848 had shaken the foundations of the old order, but the promises of liberty and equality had curdled into something darker. Louis-Napoleon Bonaparte sat uneasily on a throne built from the bones of the Republic, while in the shadows, men plotted and schemed and dreamed of the violence that would remake France according to their vision of justice.

Mary arrived in the French capital as Madame Céleste Moreau, a wealthy widow whose husband had supposedly died during the June Days uprising. Her credentials were impeccable, forged by networks of agents who had served An Dubhán for centuries, but indistinguishable from genuine documents even under the most careful scrutiny. She rented an elegant apartment overlooking the Seine, furnished it with the understated luxury that marked old money rather than new wealth, and began the careful work of inserting herself into the revolutionary circles that would shape France's future.

“The key,” An Dubhán had explained during the weeks of preparation that followed their reunion in London, “"is not to choose sides in these conflicts, but to ensure that the most useful outcomes emerge from whatever chaos ensues. Sometimes that will mean preserving leaders who serve our long-term purposes. Other times it will require eliminating those whose survival would inconvenience our plans."

The creature had provided Mary with detailed intelligence about the various factions competing for power in post-revolutionary France. She knew which republicans still dreamed of restoring the ideals of 1789, which socialists hoped to push the revolution toward more radical conclusions, which monarchists schemed to restore the Bourbon line, and which opportunists simply sought to profit from the confusion.

But more importantly, she understood how each of these groups could be manipulated through carefully applied violence. A murdered moderate could radicalize his followers. A assassinated radical could discredit his cause. A dead spy could trigger suspicions that would tear apart fragile alliances.

Her first target was Henri Delacroix, a republican journalist whose newspaper had become the voice of democratic idealism in post-revolutionary France. Delacroix was a genuine believer in the principles of liberty and equality, a man whose writings inspired hope among those who felt betrayed by the Republic's failure to deliver on its promises. An Dubhán wanted him dead, not because he was evil, but because his martyrdom would serve purposes that his continued life could not.

"Delacroix alive is merely another voice among many, the creature had explained. Delacroix dead becomes a symbol, a rallying point around which more radical elements can organise. His assassination will be blamed on monarchist agents, which will justify the kind of violent suppression that will drive moderate republicans toward more extreme positions."

Mary began attending the salons where Republican intellectuals gathered to debate the future of France. She presented herself as a woman whose loss during the uprising had given her a passionate interest in political reform, someone whose combination of wealth and widow's grief made her both attractive to men seeking funding and useful to those who needed connections among the Parisian elite.

Delacroix was immediately taken with Madame Moreau's apparent commitment to democratic principles. Here was a woman who had suffered personally under the old regime, who had lost her husband to the violence that accompanied political change, but who remained dedicated to the ideals that had justified such sacrifice. Her beauty was refined rather than flashy, her intelligence obvious but not threatening, her grief authentic enough to command sympathy while not overwhelming her other attractions.

"You understand what we're fighting for, he told her one evening after a particularly passionate discussion about press freedom and government censorship. So many of the wealthy class mouth republican slogans while secretly longing for the stability of a monarchy. But you... You've paid the price that gives your convictions substance."

Mary smiled with what appeared to be genuine warmth, though inwardly she was calculating the precise moment when Delacroix's usefulness as a living man would be exceeded by his value as a martyred symbol.

"My husband died believing that France could become something better than it had ever been," she replied, allowing her voice to carry just the right note of controlled sorrow. I cannot honour his memory by abandoning the cause he died for, regardless of how difficult the path forward might be.

Over the following weeks, Mary became Delacroix's closest confidante and, eventually, his lover. She listened to his plans for expanding his newspaper's influence, his dreams of creating a truly democratic France, his fears about the conservative forces that seemed to be regaining strength throughout Europe. She offered financial support for his publishing ventures, introductions to wealthy republicans who might fund his operations, and the kind of intimate companionship that made their professional collaboration personal as well as political.

But she also studied his routines, identified his vulnerabilities, and prepared for the moment when An Dubhán would decide that his continued existence had become counterproductive to their larger goals.

That moment came on a cold February evening when Delacroix's latest editorial had achieved exactly the kind of impact that made him too dangerous to leave alive. He had written a series of articles exposing corruption within Louis-Napoleon's government, revelations that were generating popular outrage and calls for immediate reform. The government was preparing to shut down his newspaper and arrest him for sedition, which would make him a living martyr rather than a dead symbol.

“Tonight,” An Dubhán whispered in Mary’s mind as she prepared for what would be their final evening together. “His death must appear to be the work of government agents, but the evidence must be circumstantial rather than definitive. We want suspicion and outrage, not certainty that would allow for clear retaliation.”

Mary dressed carefully for the occasion, choosing clothes that would not show bloodstains and jewellery that could be easily disposed of if it became contaminated with evidence. She met Delacroix at their usual restaurant, a small establishment in Montparnasse where republican intellectuals gathered to discuss politics over wine and simple food.

“I have wonderful news,” she told him as they settled at their customary corner table. “My banker has agreed to provide the funding you need to expand publication. Within a month, your newspaper could be reaching twice as many readers throughout France.”

Delacroix’s face lit up with excitement and gratitude. He had been struggling to keep his publication afloat despite its growing influence, and the promise of adequate funding represented the difference between survival and collapse.

“Céleste,” he said, reaching across the table to take her hand, “you cannot know what this means to me. With proper resources, we could transform the entire political landscape of France. We could create the kind of informed citizenry that democracy requires to function.”

They celebrated over dinner, planning the newspaper’s expansion and discussing the articles

Delacroix hoped to write once he was freed from financial constraints. Mary listened with apparent enthusiasm, occasionally offering suggestions that would make his work more effective while inwardly preparing for what would come next.

After dinner, they walked along the Seine toward Delacroix's apartment, their breath visible in the cold air as they continued their discussion about the future of French democracy. It was a perfect winter evening in Paris, the kind of night that made political idealism seem not just possible but inevitable.

"I keep thinking about your husband," Delacroix said as they approached his building. "About the sacrifice he made for our cause. I hope... I hope that what we're building justifies the price that people like him have paid."

"I'm sure it will," Mary replied, though she was thinking about different kinds of sacrifice and different kinds of justification than those Delacroix had in mind.

She accompanied him up to his apartment, ostensibly to review the financial documents that would formalise her support for his newspaper. But once they were alone in his study, surrounded by the books and papers that represented his life's work, Mary produced the knife she had concealed in her coat.

Delacroix's death was quick and professional, a single thrust between the ribs that pierced his heart and left him no time for cries or struggles. But Mary's work was far from finished. She spent the next hour carefully staging the scene to suggest that government agents had murdered him during a search for seditious materials, planting evidence that would point toward official involvement while leaving enough doubt to prevent definitive conclusions.

When she finally slipped away into the Paris night, Henri Delacroix's body lay among scattered papers and overturned furniture, a scene that would be discovered the next morning by his landlord and reported immediately to the police. The investigation that followed would find suggestions of government involvement but no conclusive proof, creating exactly the kind of suspicious uncertainty that An Dubhán had desired.

The reaction to Delacroix's murder was everything the ancient creature had predicted. Moderate republicans, convinced that the government had assassinated one of their most effective voices, began embracing more radical positions. Socialist leaders, seeing an opportunity to capitalise on popular outrage, called for immediate action against the forces of reaction. Even some monarchists, horrified by what appeared to be state-sponsored terrorism, began questioning their support for Louis-Napoleon's increasingly authoritarian regime.

Within weeks, the political landscape of France had shifted dramatically. The careful balance that had maintained relative stability since 1848 gave way to polarisation and radicalisation that would, in time, create the conditions for even greater upheavals.

Mary watched these developments with satisfaction, understanding for the first time the true scope of what An Dubhán had offered her. She was not just a killer, she was an architect of history, someone whose carefully applied violence could reshape entire nations according to designs that spanned decades or centuries.

"Magnificent work," the creature whispered in her mind as she planned her next assignment. ""Delacroix's death will have consequences that ripple through French politics for generations. But this is only the beginning, Mary. There are so many other threads that need to be cut or rewoven."

An Dubhán showed her visions of the future that would emerge from her work, revolutions and wars, the rise and fall of governments, the transformation of European civilisation through conflicts that would seem natural and inevitable to those who experienced them. She would be the hidden hand that guided these changes, the unseen force that determined which leaders lived and which died, which movements succeeded and which failed.

"Your next target is in Vienna," the creature informed her. "A diplomat whose survival would inconveniently stabilise the situation in Austria. His death will create the conditions for the kind of nationalist uprising that will serve our purposes perfectly."

Mary smiled as she began planning her next identity, her next approach, her next carefully orchestrated murder. She had found her true calling at last, not as a simple assassin, but as death's own ambassador to the world of politics and power.

The revolution she was creating would be unlike any that had come before. It would be subtle, sophisticated, seemingly natural in its development. But it would reshape human civilisation according to patterns that served appetites far older and more implacable than any human ambition.

Henri Delacroix had been just the first thread. There were so many others waiting to be cut.

Vienna in the spring of 1851 was a city struggling to maintain its imperial composure while nationalist fervour simmered beneath its elegant surface. The Austrian Empire had weathered the revolutionary storms of 1848, but the forces that had shaken thrones across Europe were far from spent. In the coffee houses and salons of the Habsburg capital, men spoke in careful whispers about Hungarian independence, Italian unification, and the rights of peoples to determine their own destinies.

Mary arrived as Baroness Katarina von Schwarzburg, a minor Austrian noblewoman whose family had supposedly lost their estates during the recent upheavals. Her German was flawless, her knowledge of aristocratic etiquette impeccable, her story of financial reversal common enough among the nobility to attract sympathy rather than suspicion. She took rooms at the Hotel Imperial, dressed in the understated elegance of old money temporarily reduced in circumstances, and began the delicate work of infiltrating the diplomatic circles that governed the empire's response to nationalist unrest.

Her target was Count Friedrich von Metternich, not the famous statesman who had shaped European politics for decades, but his nephew, a career diplomat whose moderate approach to nationalist demands had made him dangerously effective at defusing tensions that An Dubhán preferred to see escalate. Count Friedrich had successfully negotiated compromises in Bohemia that had prevented the kind of violent uprising that would justify harsh imperial suppression. His continued survival threatened to establish precedents that might spread to other restive provinces.

“Von Metternich understands the art of strategic concession,” An Dubhán had explained during Mary’s preparation in Paris. “He gives nationalist movements just enough of what they want to prevent them from pursuing more radical goals. His death must appear to be the work of extremist elements, either German nationalists who see him as too sympathetic to Slavic demands, or Slavic radicals who view his compromises as inadequate half-measures.”

Mary studied her target through the social mechanisms of Viennese high society. Count Friedrich was a widower in his fifties, intelligent and cultured, possessed of the kind of world-weary sophistication that came from decades of diplomatic service. He had no children, few close friends, and a reputation for discretion that made him valuable to the government and attractive to women who appreciated both intellect and mystery in their companions.

She encountered him at a reception hosted by the French ambassador, one of those glittering affairs where the representatives of various powers gathered to conduct the real business of diplomacy beneath a veneer of social pleasantry. Count Friedrich was discussing the situation in Hungary with a group of fellow diplomats, his voice carrying the calm authority of someone accustomed to navigating complex political currents.

“The key to managing nationalist sentiment,” he was saying as Mary approached their circle, “is to understand that it represents genuine grievances that cannot be dismissed through force alone. People who feel heard and respected are far less likely to resort to violence than those who believe their concerns are being ignored."

Mary introduced herself to the group with the practiced grace of someone born to such gatherings, allowing her beauty and apparent vulnerability to capture the attention of men who spent their days dealing with abstract political problems rather than flesh-and-blood human needs."Baroness von Schwarzburg," Count Friedrich said with genuine interest as they were introduced. "I believe I knew your late father, Count Wilhelm, was it not? A tragic loss during the difficulties in Bohemia."

"Indeed," Mary replied, though no such person had ever existed. An Dubhán's agents had crafted her fictional background with meticulous attention to detail, creating a family history that would withstand casual investigation while explaining her presence in Vienna and her interest in political affairs.

Over the following weeks, Mary and Count Friedrich developed the kind of relationship that Vienna's diplomatic community expected between an attractive widow and an eligible bachelor of appropriate social standing. They attended the same receptions, shared boxes at the opera, and took walks in the Prater while discussing the philosophical foundations of governance and the challenges of managing diverse populations within a single empire.

Count Friedrich was genuinely attracted to Mary's apparent combination of beauty and intelligence, but he was also intrigued by her perspective on the nationalist question. As someone who had supposedly lost family property due to ethnic violence, she brought a personal dimension to discussions that were usually conducted in abstract terms.

"You understand the human cost of political upheaval," he told her one evening as they dined at Sacher's, the famous hotel where Vienna's elite gathered to see and be seen. "Too many of my colleagues treat these issues as chess problems to be solved through clever manoeuvring, but you've experienced firsthand what happens when diplomacy fails."

Mary nodded thoughtfully, her expression conveying the kind of hard-won wisdom that personal tragedy supposedly provided. "Perhaps that's why I find your approach so refreshing, Friedrich. You seem to understand that behind every political demand are real people with real needs, real fears, real hopes for their children's futures."

She was building toward the moment when her fictional perspective would provide the justification for his death. An Dubhán had crafted an elegant scenario in which Count Friedrich's murder would appear to be the work of extremists who viewed his moderate approach as betrayal, either German radicals who saw his concessions to Slavic demands as treason, or Slavic revolutionaries who considered his compromises insufficient.

The opportunity came when Count Friedrich confided his plans for a secret meeting with Hungarian nationalist leaders in Budapest. He hoped to negotiate another of his strategic compromises, offering the Hungarians enough autonomy to satisfy moderate elements within their movement while maintaining Habsburg authority over the broader empire.

"It's dangerous work," he admitted to Mary as they walked along the Danube, watching the spring ice break apart and flow toward the distant Black Sea. "There are elements on both sides who prefer confrontation to compromise, who see any negotiation as weakness or betrayal. But I believe that reasonable people can find solutions that serve everyone's essential interests."

Mary listened with apparent concern, her expression conveying both admiration for his courage and fear for his safety. "Perhaps you should take additional security precautions," she suggested. "If there are extremists who oppose what you're trying to accomplish..."

"I've considered that," Count Friedrich replied, "but too much security would signal the importance of the meeting to precisely the people we're trying to avoid alerting. Sometimes discretion requires accepting certain risks."

That evening, Mary sent coded messages through An Dubhán's network, arranging for assets to be positioned in Budapest while she prepared for her own journey to the Hungarian capital. Count Friedrich's death would need to be choreographed with particular care, it must appear spontaneous while actually being precisely orchestrated, must seem like the work of local extremists while leaving enough ambiguous evidence to prevent definitive conclusions about which faction was responsible.

She accompanied Count Friedrich to Budapest as his unofficial consort, a role that provided perfect cover for her presence while ensuring that she would have intimate access to his person at the crucial moment. They travelled by private carriage, staying at discreet inns along the way, their journey having all the appearances of a romantic getaway rather than a diplomatic mission.

The meeting was scheduled to take place in a private room at the Hotel Europa, one of Budapest's finest establishments, where Hungarian nobles and German officials could encounter each other without attracting unwanted attention. Count Friedrich had arranged to meet with three moderate Hungarian leaders who shared his belief that compromise offered a better path forward than continued confrontation.

Mary had studied the hotel's layout during their first evening in Budapest, identifying escape routes and timing the movements of staff and guests. An Dubhán's local agents had provided her with detailed intelligence about the Hungarian participants in the meeting, including information about their personal habits and political vulnerabilities that would be crucial for staging the aftermath of Count Friedrich's death.

The murder itself was almost anticlimactic after so much careful preparation. Mary waited until Count Friedrich had retired to his room after the successful conclusion of his negotiations, then visited him under the pretence of celebrating their apparent success. The poison she administered was one that would cause symptoms resembling a heart attack brought on by excitement, appropriate for a diplomat who had just concluded delicate negotiations under considerable stress.

But the real artistry came in the hours that followed, as Mary worked with An Dubhán's agents to create the impression that radical Hungarian nationalists had assassinated the Austrian diplomat in response to his moderate policies. Evidence was planted suggesting that extremist elements had viewed the compromise negotiations as betrayal of Hungarian independence aspirations, while other clues pointed toward German radicals who saw Count Friedrich's concessions as treasonous weakness..

When Count Friedrich;s body was discovered the next morning, the investigation that followed found exactly the kind of contradictory evidence that An Dubhán had desired. Hungarian authorities suspected German agents, German officials blamed Hungarian extremists, and moderate elements on both sides began questioning whether compromise was possible with such radical opposition.

The careful balance that Count Friedrich had spent years constructing began to collapse within weeks of his death. Hungarian moderates, convinced that Austrian extremists had murdered their diplomatic partner, moved toward more radical positions. German officials, believing that Hungarian radicals had assassinated their negotiator, adopted harsher policies toward nationalist demands.

The spiral toward confrontation that An Dubhán had orchestrated would eventually culminate in exactly the kind of violent uprising that would justify massive imperial suppression, creating the cycles of repression and rebellion that fed the ancient creature’s hunger while reshaping the political landscape of Central Europe according to its purposes.

Mary watched these developments unfold with growing appreciation for the sophisticated nature of the work she was doing. Each death created ripple effects that extended far beyond the immediate political consequences, shaping the attitudes and expectations of entire populations in ways that would influence their behavior for generations.

“You’re beginning to understand the true scope of what we’'re accomplishing,” An Dubhán observed as Mary prepared to leave Vienna for her next assignment. “Individual murders are merely tools, Mary. What we’re really doing is surgery on the body politic of human civilisation itself.”The creature showed her visions of the future that would emerge from her work, wars and revolutions that would seem inevitable to those who experienced them, but which were actually the carefully orchestrated results of strategic assassinations performed decades earlier. She was not just killing individuals; she was killing possibilities, eliminating the moderate voices that might have prevented conflicts and preserving the extremist elements that would make such conflicts inevitable.

“Where next?"” Mary asked, though she was already anticipating the answer.

“Italy,"” An Dubhán replied with satisfaction.”

“The situation there requires the kind of delicate touch that only you can provide. There are several key figures whose continued survival would inconvenience our plans for Italian unification, which must happen, but happen in precisely the right way to serve our longer-term purposes."”

Mary smiled as she began planning her next identity, her next approach, her next contribution to the reshaping of European civilisation. She had found work worthy of her talents at last, not simple murder, but murder as statecraft, assassination as historical artistry.

The revolution she was creating would be unlike any that had come before, precisely because those who experienced it would never understand that it was being created at all.

Chapter Seventeen
The Italian Gambit

Rome in the autumn of 1852 was a city caught between the weight of ancient history and the pull of modern ambition. The Papal States struggled to maintain their temporal authority while nationalist fervour swept across the Italian peninsula, promising unity under secular leadership that would reduce the Pope to a purely spiritual role. In the shadowed corridors of the Vatican and the sun-drenched piazzas where Roman citizens gathered to discuss the future, the tension between tradition and revolution crackled like electricity before a storm.

Mary arrived as Contessa Elena Ravenna, a Venetian noblewoman whose family had supposedly fled Austrian rule during the recent upheavals in the north. Her Italian was perfect, her knowledge of regional dialects and customs encyclopedic, her story of exile and loss designed to evoke sympathy while explaining her presence in the Papal capital. She rented a palazzo near the Spanish Steps, furnished it with the careful elegance that spoke of old wealth temporarily reduced in circumstances, and began the delicate work of positioning herself within the complex web of Italian politics.

An Dubhán had provided her with detailed intelligence about the various forces competing to shape

Italy's future. She understood the vision of Giuseppe Mazzini, the republican idealist who dreamed of a unified Italian nation governed by democratic principles. She knew the ambitions of Count Camillo di Cavour, the Piedmontese statesman who sought unity under Sardinian leadership. She was familiar with Giuseppe Garibaldi's military genius and his commitment to popular liberation, and she comprehended the delicate position of Pope Pius IX, who found himself torn between his spiritual mission and his role as a temporal ruler.

But more importantly, she understood how each of these figures could serve An Dubhán's purposes, not as they intended, but as instruments in a larger symphony of controlled chaos that would reshape Italian civilisation according to patterns the ancient creature had been orchestrating for centuries.

"The key to the Italian situation," An Dubhán had explained during her preparation in Vienna, "is ensuring that unification occurs, but occurs in a manner that maximises conflict rather than resolving it. A united Italy governed by moderate voices who understand the value of compromise would be of little use to us. But a united Italy born from violence and maintained through suppression of regional differences, that would provide the kind of ongoing tension that feeds our purposes."

Her first target was Cardinal Alessandro Antonelli, the Pope's Secretary of State and one of the most influential voices in the Vatican's response to Italian nationalism. Cardinal Antonelli was a pragmatic man who understood that the Church's temporal power was doomed, but who hoped to negotiate a transition that would preserve papal spiritual authority while acknowledging secular political realities. His diplomatic skills had already prevented several confrontations that might have escalated into open warfare between papal forces and nationalist armies.

"Antonelli alive represents the possibility of peaceful transition," the creature had observed. "His death will eliminate the moderate voice within the Vatican that might have prevented the kind of confrontation we require. Without his influence, Pope Pius IX will be left to rely on advisors who favour resistance over accommodation."

Mary began attending the salons where Roman intellectuals gathered to debate the future of the peninsula. She presented herself as a woman whose family's suffering under Austrian rule had given her a passionate commitment to Italian independence, but whose aristocratic background made her sensitive to the legitimate concerns of those who feared that unity might come at the cost of regional traditions and religious authority.

Cardinal Antonelli was immediately impressed by Contessa Ravenna's apparent combination of political sophistication and spiritual devotion. Here was a woman who understood the complexities of the Italian situation, who recognised that the Church's interests were not necessarily opposed to national unification, who might serve as a bridge between secular and religious approaches to the challenges that faced the peninsula.

"You speak with rare wisdom, Contessa," he told her after a particularly nuanced discussion about the relationship between temporal and spiritual authority. "Too many people see this as a simple choice between tradition and progress, between faith and reason. But you understand that the Church's mission transcends political arrangements, that we can serve God effectively under any form of government that respects religious liberty.

Mary nodded thoughtfully, her expression conveying the kind of deep reflection that comes from personal experience with the costs of political upheaval. "My family's suffering taught me that rigid positions often produce outcomes that serve no one's interests," she replied. "Perhaps there are paths forward that honour both our spiritual heritage and our political aspirations."

Over the following weeks, Mary became Cardinal Antonelli's most trusted confidante among the Roman laity. She listened to his plans for negotiating with nationalist leaders, his vision of a future Italian state that would respect papal spiritual authority while acknowledging secular political realities, his careful strategies for managing the transition from the old order to whatever new arrangements might emerge.

But she also studied his routines, identified his vulnerabilities, and prepared for the moment when An Dubhán would decide that his influence had become counterproductive to their larger goals.

That moment came when Cardinal Antonelli's latest diplomatic initiative threatened to achieve exactly the kind of peaceful resolution that the ancient creature wanted to prevent. He had opened secret negotiations with representatives of the Piedmontese government, discussions that might lead to a concordat defining the Church's role in a unified Italian state. Such an agreement would eliminate the pretext for the violent confrontation that An Dubhán required.

"Tonight," the creature whispered in Mary's mind as she prepared for what would be their final meeting. "His death must appear to be the work of radical republicans who view any accommodation with the Church as a betrayal of secular principles. We need the Vatican to believe that moderate nationalism is impossible, that they face enemies who will accept nothing less than the complete destruction of papal authority.

Mary dressed carefully for the occasion, choosing clothes that would not restrict her movement and could be easily disposed of if they became contaminated with evidence. She met Cardinal Antonelli at his private study in the Vatican, ostensibly to discuss a charitable foundation she wished to establish in memory of her fictional family members who had died during the Austrian occupation of Venice.

"Your generosity honours both their memory and the Church"s mission,"" Cardinal Antonelli said as they reviewed the papers she had prepared for the meeting. "Such foundations can serve as bridges between secular wealth and spiritual purpose, demonstrating that the Church's role in modern society need not be diminished by political change."

They discussed the details of the charitable work she proposed, the ways in which such initiatives might serve as models for cooperation between the Church and whatever secular government might emerge from Italian unification. Cardinal Antonelli was genuinely excited by the possibilities, seeing in Mary's proposal exactly the kind of constructive engagement that could ease the transition to new political arrangements.

The poison she administered was absorbed through his skin as he handled the documents she had prepared, a substance that would cause symptoms resembling the heart failure that might be expected in an elderly man working under considerable stress. But Marys work extended far beyond the simple act of murder.

After Cardinal Antonelli's death, she spent several hours carefully staging evidence that would point toward radical republican involvement. She planted materials suggesting that extremist elements viewed any negotiation with the Vatican as a betrayal of secular principles, that they preferred violent confrontation to peaceful resolution of Church-state tensions.

When Cardinal Antonelli's body was discovered the next morning by his secretary, the investigation that followed found exactly the kind of circumstantial evidence that An Dubhán had desired. The Vatican was convinced that radical republicans had assassinated their most skilled negotiator, while nationalist leaders suspected that reactionary forces within the Church had eliminated their most reasonable interlocutor.

The careful diplomatic balance that Cardinal Antonelli had spent years constructing collapsed within days of his death. Pope Pius IX, deprived of his most trusted advisor's moderating influence, began listening to hardline Cardinals who favored resistance over accommodation. Nationalist leaders, convinced that the Church would never accept secular authority, abandoned hopes for peaceful transition and began preparing for the kind of violent confrontation that would justify harsh suppression of religious institutions.

Mary watched these developments with satisfaction, understanding that she had eliminated not just an individual but an entire approach to managing political change. Cardinal Antonelli's death had removed the possibility of compromise, ensuring that Italian unification would be achieved through conflict rather than negotiation.

But her work in Rome was far from finished. An Dubhán had identified several other key figures whose survival might interfere with the creature's plans for controlling the manner and consequences of Italian unity. Each would require different methods, different approaches, different kinds of evidence to ensure that their deaths served the larger purpose of maximizing rather than minimizing conflict.

Her next target was Count Giuseppe Pasolini, a moderate nationalist leader whose influence with both secular and religious authorities made him dangerously effective at building bridges between opposing factions. His assassination would need to be attributed to conservative elements who opposed any form of national unity, creating the kind of martyrdom that would radicalise moderate nationalists while providing justification for more extreme measures.

After Pasolini, she would turn her attention to Monsignor Giacomo Margotti, an influential Church journalist whose writings had begun advocating for accommodation with nationalist aspirations. His death would eliminate another moderate voice within the Vatican while creating suspicions that secular authorities were systematically targeting religious leaders.

Each murder would be carefully choreographed to maximise the polarisation of Italian society, eliminating the moderate voices that might have prevented violent confrontation while preserving the extremist elements that would make such confrontation inevitable. By the time Mary finished her work in Italy, the peninsula would be unified , but unified through bloodshed that would poison the new nation's political culture for generations to come.

"You're creating a masterpiece," An Dubhán observed as Mary planned her next series of assassinations. +"Not just individual deaths, but a systematic elimination of the possibility of peaceful progress. When Italian unity finally comes, it will be built on the foundations of violence and suspicion that will serve our purposes for decades."

Mary smiled as she began preparing her approach to Count Pasolini. She had found work that challenged every aspect of her skills, not just as a killer, but as a student of human nature, a manipulator of political forces, an artist whose medium was the raw material of history itself.

The Italian gambit was proceeding exactly as planned. Soon, the entire peninsula would be convulsed by exactly the kind of violence that An Dubhán required, conflicts that would seem inevitable to those who experienced them but which were actually the carefully orchestrated results of strategic murders performed by a woman who had learned to see individual deaths as brush strokes in a much larger painting.

And Italy was only the beginning. Europe was full of moderate voices that needed to be silenced, reasonable people whose very reasonableness made them obstacles to the ancient creature's vision of controlled chaos.

Chapter Eighteen
Blood and Unity

The assassination of Count Giuseppe Pasolini proved more challenging than Mary had anticipated. Unlike Cardinal Antonelli, who had been vulnerable due to his position within the Vatican's hierarchical structure, Pasolini was a secular nobleman who moved freely through Roman society and maintained extensive security arrangements developed during years of political activism. He had survived three previous assassination attempts by various extremist factions, and his wariness made casual approaches nearly impossible.

Mary spent weeks studying his patterns, learning that Pasolini's one weakness was his devotion to his teenage daughter, Maria, who had been born with a progressive illness that required constant medical attention. The Count's love for his child was absolute, and he would interrupt any political activity to respond to her needs. It was through this paternal vulnerability that Mary found her opening.

She arranged to be introduced to the Pasolini household as Dr. Catherine Brennan, an Irish physician who had studied advanced treatments for degenerative diseases at the medical colleges of Edinburgh and Vienna. Her credentials, forged by An Dubhán's network, were impressive enough to convince the desperate father that she might offer hope where Italian doctors had provided only grim prognoses.

"Dr. Brennan," Count Pasolini said when they first met in his daughter's sickroom, "I have consulted with every medical authority in Rome, and they all tell me that Maria's condition is beyond treatment. But your letter suggested that there might be new approaches developed in northern European hospitals."

Mary examined the pale, thin girl who lay propped against silk pillows, noting the symptoms that she recognized from An Dubhán's extensive knowledge of human pathology. Maria Pasolini was indeed dying, though more slowly than her father feared. Her condition was degenerative but not immediately fatal, she might have years of increasingly limited life ahead of her.

"There are experimental treatments," Mary said carefully, "that have shown promise in similar cases. Nothing I can guarantee, you understand, but approaches that might slow the progression of her illness or even achieve some improvement in her symptoms."

The hope that flared in Count Pasolini's eyes was painful to witness. Here was a man who had dedicated his life to the liberation of Italy, who had risked everything for political principles, but who would abandon all of it if he could somehow save his daughter's life.

Over the following weeks, Mary became a fixture in the Pasolini household, administering treatments that provided just enough improvement in Maria's condition to convince her father that recovery might be possible. The medicines she used were genuine, An Dubhán's knowledge extended to healing as well as harming, but they were palliative rather than curative, designed to create the illusion of progress while the underlying disease continued its inexorable advance.

But Mary's real purpose was not medical care but intelligence gathering. As Dr. Brennan, she gained access to Count Pasolini's private study, where she observed his correspondence with moderate leaders throughout Italy and learned the details of his plans for achieving unity through negotiated settlement rather than armed revolution.

"The tragedy of our situation," Pasolini confided to her one evening as they discussed Maria's treatment, "is that both sides want essentially the same thing, a unified Italy that honors both our national aspirations and our spiritual heritage. The Church fears that unification means the destruction of religious authority, while nationalists worry that accommodation with Rome means betraying secular principles. But these are not irreconcilable positions if reasonable people are willing to compromise."

Mary listened with apparent sympathy while inwardly calculating how much damage his reasonable approach could do to An Dubhán's plans. Pasolini was precisely the kind of moderate voice that could prevent the violent confrontation the ancient creature required. His death would need to be attributed to extremist elements who viewed any compromise as betrayal.

The opportunity came when Maria's condition suddenly worsened, not due to her underlying disease, but because of a complication that Mary had carefully induced through subtle adjustments to her treatment regimen. The girl developed a severe fever that appeared to be a natural progression of her illness but which Mary knew would prove fatal within days.

Count Pasolini was devastated by this apparent failure of the experimental treatment that had offered such hope. He spent every moment at his daughter's bedside, abandoning his political activities to focus entirely on her care. It was during one of these long vigils that Mary struck.

"Count," she said as they sat in the darkened sickroom, watching Maria struggle with each labored breath, "I'm afraid I must tell you something that will be difficult to hear. The complications your daughter is experiencing, they're not entirely natural."

Pasolini looked up from his daughter's bedside with the hollow eyes of a man who had already lost everything that mattered to him. "What do you mean?"

"I've discovered evidence that someone has been interfering with her treatment," Mary said, her voice carrying the kind of reluctant honesty that made terrible news believable. "Someone with access to this house, someone who wanted to ensure that the experimental therapy failed."

The count's face went white as the implications of her words sank in. "Who? Who would do such a thing?"

Mary produced documents she had carefully prepared, papers that suggested Austrian agents had infiltrated the household specifically to ensure that Pasolini's moderate approach to Italian unification would be discredited. The evidence pointed toward a sophisticated operation designed to eliminate key nationalist leaders through their personal vulnerabilities rather than direct assassination.

"They knew that killing you outright would make you a martyr," Mary explained as Pasolini examined the forged papers with shaking hands. "But destroying your daughter while making it appear to be a failure of foreign medical treatment, that would break your spirit while discrediting the international connections that make your diplomatic approach possible."

Count Pasolini's grief transformed into rage as he absorbed what appeared to be proof that his daughter's death had been engineered by Austria's secret police. The moderate politician who had always advocated for peaceful solutions suddenly found himself consumed by hatred for those who would use a child's life as a weapon in their political calculations.

"What can be done?" he asked, his voice hoarse with emotion. "Can Maria be saved?"

"I'm afraid it's too late for that," Mary said with apparent regret. "The poison they've been administering has progressed too far. But we can ensure that her death is not in vain, that the people responsible face justice for what they've done."

She spent the next hour carefully guiding Pasolini toward the conclusion she wanted him to reach, that the only appropriate response to such monstrous cruelty was violent retaliation against Austrian interests throughout Italy. The moderate leader who had spent years advocating for diplomatic solutions became convinced that negotiation was impossible with enemies who would murder children to achieve political goals.

Count Pasolini died two days later, shot down in the street as he led an attack on the Austrian embassy in Rome. His assassination was carried out by An Dubhán's agents posing as Austrian security personnel, creating exactly the kind of martyrdom that would radicalize moderate nationalists while providing justification for Austrian military intervention.

But the real masterpiece was the story that emerged from his death. Maria Pasolini's suffering became a symbol of Austrian cruelty, proof that the empire would stop at nothing to prevent Italian unity. The moderate leader who had advocated for compromise was transformed into a hero who had died fighting against enemies too evil to deserve mercy.

"Elegant work," An Dubhán observed as Mary prepared to leave the Pasolini household for the final time. "You didn't just eliminate a moderate voice, you converted him into an argument for extremism. His death will inspire exactly the kind of violent nationalism that serves our purposes."

Mary nodded with satisfaction as she began planning her approach to Monsignor Margotti. Each assassination was becoming more sophisticated, more perfectly calibrated to achieve multiple objectives simultaneously. She was not just killing individuals but transforming the entire political landscape of Italy through carefully orchestrated tragedies that appeared natural while serving purposes that no human observer could comprehend.

The unification of Italy would happen, just as An Dubhán had predicted. But it would happen through blood and betrayal, through the systematic elimination of every voice that might have counseled moderation or compromise. When the new nation finally emerged, it would be built on foundations of violence and suspicion that would serve the ancient creature's purposes for generations to come.

Monsignor Margotti's death would complete the Italian phase of Mary's work, eliminating the last significant moderate voice within the Church hierarchy while creating the conditions for the kind of violent confrontation between secular and religious authorities that would poison Italian politics for decades.

And after Italy, there would be Germany, where Bismarck's ambitions for Prussian dominance could be channeled in directions that served An Dubhán's vision of controlled chaos. After Germany, there would be Russia, where the Tsarist system's internal contradictions could be exploited to create the kind of revolutionary upheaval that would reshape Eastern Europe according to patterns the ancient creature had been orchestrating since the dawn of human civilization.

Mary Costello had found her true calling at last, not as a simple killer, but as an architect of history itself, a sculptor whose medium was human ambition and whose finished works were the wars and revolutions that would define the modern world.

Chapter Nineteen
The Final Thread

Monsignor Giacomo Margotti was a different kind of target than Mary had eliminated before. Where Cardinal Antonelli had been a diplomat and Count Pasolini a politician, Margotti was fundamentally a scholar, a man whose power came not from institutional position but from the force of his ideas. His weekly journal, *L'Armonia della Fede e della Ragione*, had become the most influential Catholic publication in Italy, read by priests and laymen alike who struggled to understand how their faith could coexist with the nationalist aspirations sweeping across the peninsula.

Margotti's writings had begun advocating for what he called "patriotic Catholicism", the idea that love of country and devotion to the Church were not contradictory impulses but complementary aspects of a properly formed Christian conscience. His theology was sophisticated enough to convince conservative clergy while remaining accessible to ordinary believers, and his political analysis demonstrated that Italian unity need not mean the destruction of papal authority.

"Margotti is the most dangerous kind of moderate," An Dubhán had explained as Mary prepared for her final assignment in Italy. "His influence comes not from political position but from intellectual authority. Politicians can be discredited through scandal or eliminated through assassination, but ideas require more sophisticated forms of destruction."

The creature's strategy for dealing with Margotti was characteristically elegant. Rather than simply killing him, Mary would orchestrate his corruption, transforming the moderate voice that advocated for accommodation into a radical one that preached holy war against secular authority. The death of his ideas would be more valuable than the death of his body.

Mary approached him through his weakness for intellectual discourse. She appeared at a theological conference in Florence as Sister Agatha McKenna, an Irish nun whose convent had supposedly been destroyed during the recent upheavals in her homeland. Her credentials identified her as a scholar of Church history with particular expertise in the relationship between temporal and spiritual authority during periods of political change.

Monsignor Margotti was immediately intrigued by Sister Agatha's perspective on the Irish situation. Here was a woman whose firsthand experience with violent nationalism provided a valuable counterpoint to the Italian situation, someone who could speak authoritatively about what happened when accommodation between Church and secular authority proved impossible.

"Tell me, Sister," he said during one of their first conversations, "how did the Church in Ireland respond to the failed rebellions of recent decades? Were there attempts at the kind of patriotic synthesis that I've been advocating for our Italian situation?"

Mary spoke eloquently about fictional efforts by Irish clergy to support nationalist aspirations while maintaining loyalty to Rome, painting a picture of moderate voices who had tried to bridge the gap between religious devotion and political independence. But she also described, with apparent sadness, how such efforts had ultimately failed in the face of English intransigence and radical nationalist impatience.

"The tragedy," she said with the kind of weary wisdom that comes from witnessing repeated failures, "was that reasonable people on both sides wanted essentially the same thing, a Catholic Ireland that could govern itself while remaining spiritually united with Rome. But the extremists on both sides preferred conflict to compromise, and eventually they succeeded in making accommodation impossible."

Over the following weeks, Mary became Margotti's closest confidante and collaborator. She helped him research historical precedents for Church-state cooperation, contributed articles to his journal that demonstrated the compatibility between Catholic teaching and national sovereignty, and participated in the theological discussions that shaped his thinking about the future of Italian Catholicism.

But she also began introducing subtle distortions into their work together, small modifications to historical examples, carefully selected quotations that supported more radical conclusions than their original contexts had intended, theological arguments that pushed Margotti's thinking in directions he might not have pursued on his own.

"I've been studying the early Christian communities," she told him during one of their research sessions, "and I'm struck by how often compromise with secular authority led to corruption of the Church's essential mission. Perhaps there are some political arrangements that are simply incompatible with authentic Christian witness."

The process of corrupting Margotti's thinking required months of patient work. Mary could not simply argue for radical positions, that would have triggered his intellectual defenses and made him suspicious of her motives. Instead, she had to lead him gradually toward conclusions that seemed to emerge naturally from his own research and reflection.

She provided him with documents that appeared to prove that moderate Catholic leaders in other countries had been systematically betrayed by secular governments they had trusted. She arranged for him to meet with witnesses whose testimony suggested that accommodation with nationalist movements inevitably led to restrictions on religious freedom. She guided his attention toward theological sources that emphasized the Church's prophetic role in confronting worldly power rather than cooperating with it.

The transformation was subtle but unmistakable. Margotti's writings gradually shifted from advocating patriotic Catholicism to warning about the dangers of secular nationalism. His journal began publishing articles that questioned whether Italian unity was compatible with authentic Catholic faith. His theological position evolved from supporting accommodation to demanding that the

Church resist any compromise with forces that threatened its spiritual authority.

"I fear I've been naive," Margotti confided to Mary during one of their final conversations in his study. "I wanted to believe that reasonable people could find solutions that honored both faith and patriotism. But the evidence you've helped me discover suggests that such accommodations have historically led to the corruption of the Church's mission and the betrayal of its fundamental principles."

Mary nodded with apparent sadness, though inwardly she was calculating the broader implications of his intellectual transformation. Margotti's conversion to a more radical position would eliminate the most influential moderate voice within Italian Catholicism while providing theological justification for the kind of violent confrontation that An Dubhán required.

"Perhaps," she suggested gently, "your earlier writings were not wrong but premature. Maybe the kind of synthesis you advocated will be possible in the future, after the Church has demonstrated its willingness to defend its essential principles against secular encroachment."

But Mary's work was not yet complete. Converting Margotti from moderate to radical was only the first step in An Dubhán's plan. The second step required his destruction in a manner that would discredit radical Catholicism while simultaneously eliminating the intellectual framework he had developed.

The opportunity came when Margotti's transformed writings began attracting attention from secular authorities who viewed his new positions as dangerously inflammatory. His journal was placed under government surveillance, and there were rumors that he might face charges of sedition for encouraging Catholic resistance to Italian unification.

Mary used her network of contacts to arrange for evidence of Margotti's "treason" to be discovered by government agents, correspondence that appeared to show him coordinating with Austrian intelligence services, financial records that suggested he was being paid to oppose Italian unity, documents that portrayed his theological arguments as cover for foreign subversion.

The raid on Margotti's residence was swift and thorough. Government agents found exactly the evidence they had been led to expect, material that portrayed the respected theologian as a foreign agent whose religious arguments masked treasonous activities. Margotti was arrested, tried, and executed within a month, a process that shocked Italian Catholics who had respected his scholarship and terrified moderate clergy who understood that they too might face similar accusations.

But the real masterpiece was the aftermath of his death. The evidence that had justified Margotti's execution was gradually revealed to be fabricated, creating the impression that secular authorities had murdered an innocent priest to silence religious opposition to their political goals. The martyr they had created became a symbol of government persecution of the Church, while his radical writings provided theological justification for violent resistance to secular authority.

"Perfect," An Dubhán observed as Mary prepared to leave Italy for her next assignment. "You have eliminated both moderate accommodation and intellectual radicalism with a single operation. Margotti's death will inspire exactly the kind of mindless violence that serves our purposes while discrediting the kind of thoughtful opposition that might have posed a real threat to secular authority."

Mary smiled as she watched the riots that erupted in Rome following news of Margotti's execution. Catholic mobs attacked government buildings while secular authorities responded with the kind of harsh suppression that would justify even more extreme measures. The careful balance between faith and patriotism that might have made Italian unification a peaceful process had been destroyed, replaced by the mutual hatred and suspicion that would poison Italian politics for generations.

Her work in Italy was complete. The peninsula would indeed be unified, just as the nationalist leaders desired. But it would be unified through violence and maintained through oppression, exactly as An Dubhán had planned. The moderate voices that might have created a different kind of future had been systematically eliminated, leaving only extremists whose conflicts would feed the ancient creature's hunger while serving its larger purposes.

"Where next?" Mary asked, though she was already anticipating the answer.

"Germany," An Dubhán replied with satisfaction. "Bismarck's ambitions for Prussian hegemony provide excellent opportunities for the kind of controlled chaos we specialize in creating. There are several key figures whose elimination will ensure that German unification follows the pattern we require, violent, divisive, and ultimately unstable."

Mary nodded as she began planning her next identity, her next approach to the systematic reshaping of European civilization. She had learned to think in decades rather than years, to see individual assassinations as part of larger patterns that would influence human development for generations.

The Italian gambit had been a complete success. Now it was time to apply the same principles to the German situation, to ensure that the emergence of a unified German state would create the kind of European balance of power that would make future conflicts inevitable.

She was no longer just Mary Costello, Irish murderess. She had become something far more significant, An Dubhán's agent in the world of human ambition, a sculptor of history whose medium was violence and whose finished works were the wars and revolutions that would define the modern age.

Chapter Twenty
Back to Where It All Began

The cottage still stood beside the bog, though forty years of Irish weather had reduced it to little more than a shell of crumbling stone and rotting thatch. Mary stood at the edge of the property where she had been born, where she had learned the taste of hunger and the weight of her father's fists, where she had buried the bodies of her family in unmarked graves that were now indistinguishable from the wild growth that had reclaimed the land.

She had returned to Ireland as herself for the first time since her execution, not as Lady Sanguinaire or Sister Magdalene or Contessa Ravenna, but as Mary Costello, come home to the place where her story had begun. An Dubhán had granted her this pilgrimage, though the ancient creature's reasons remained characteristically opaque.

"Every instrument requires periodic maintenance," it had said when she expressed her need to return to these origins. "Even the finest tools can lose their edge if they are not properly cared for. Go home, Mary. Remember what you are beneath all the identities you have worn. Restore yourself to the simplicity that made you so effective."

The village of Ballymore had grown smaller rather than larger during the decades of her absence. The famine had taken its toll here as everywhere else in Ireland, emptying cottages and forcing families to seek better fortunes in America or Australia or the cities of England. Those who remained eked out the same marginal existence that had characterized rural Irish life for centuries, scratching sustenance from soil that yielded little more than stones and sorrow.

Mary walked through streets she had known as a child, noting the changes that time had wrought while marveling at how much remained exactly as she remembered it. The church where Father O'Brien had once preached still stood, though a younger priest now tended its small congregation. The pub where her father had drunk away what little money the family possessed still served the same harsh whiskey to the same kind of desperate men. The well where she had been drawing water when Padraig attacked her still provided the village's most reliable source of clean water.

But it was not nostalgia that had brought Mary back to this place. She had come because something was calling to her, something that had been growing stronger the further she traveled from the centers of European power where she had been working. It was a pull she felt in her bones, a recognition that her work of reshaping human civilization through strategic murder was approaching some kind of culmination that required her presence at the scene of her first killing.

She found the grove of oak trees where she had struck down her brother with that stone so many years ago. The trees had grown larger, their branches now forming a canopy so thick that the ground beneath them remained in perpetual twilight. But the clearing where Padraig had tried to rape her, where she had discovered her capacity for violence, where her long partnership with An Dubhán had truly begun, that space remained exactly as she remembered it.

Mary knelt beside the spot where she had buried her brother's body, her fingers tracing the outline of earth that had long since settled into the natural contours of the forest floor. There was no marker, no indication that a human being lay beneath this unremarkable patch of ground. Padraig Costello had vanished from the world as completely as if he had never existed.

“I've become everything you feared I might,” she said aloud to the grave, though she was not sure if she was addressing her brother’s spirit or simply the memory of what he had represented. "Everything you tried to turn me into through your cruelty. You wanted me to understand that I was powerless, that I existed only to serve the needs of those stronger than myself. Instead, you taught me that power comes to those willing to take it, regardless of the cost.”

The grove was silent except for the whisper of wind through leaves that had turned golden with the approach of autumn. But Mary could feel something stirring in the shadows between the trees, a presence that had been waiting for her return with the patience of stone.

An Dubhán emerged from the darkness between the oak trunks, its form more solid and substantial than she had ever seen it. The creature appeared almost human in the dim light of the grove, though its eyes held depths that belonged to no earthly being and its smile revealed knowledge that predated human civilisation.

“Welcome home, Mary,” it said, settling itself on a fallen log as if it were a traveller resting after a long journey. "How does it feel to return to the place where you first tasted blood, where you first understood what you were truly capable of becoming?”

Mary looked around the grove, remembering the terrified girl who had fought for her life in this place, who had struck down her rapist brother and felt the world shift around her as she crossed the line between victim and killer.

“Different than I expected, she admitted. “Smaller. Less significant. I remember it as the centre of the universe, the place where everything changed. But now it seems like just another patch of Irish wilderness where violence happened to occur.”

“That is because you have grown beyond this place,”. An Dubhán observed. “When you killed Padraig here, you were a frightened child reacting to an immediate threat. Now you are something far more sophisticated, an architect of historical change, a sculptor whose medium is human ambition itself. This grove was your nursery, Mary. The battlefields of Europe have been your university."

The creature rose from its resting place and began to walk slowly around the clearing, its movements stirring memories that Mary had thought buried beneath decades of assumed identities and strategic murders.

"But nurseries have their own importance," it continued. "They are where we learn the fundamental lessons that shape everything that comes after. What did you learn here, Mary, in this place where your education truly began?"

Mary considered the question, her mind traveling back to that moment of violent transformation when she had felt her brother's blood on her hands and understood for the first time that she was capable of taking life.

"That I was not powerless," she said finally. "That I could choose to be the one who lived rather than the one who died. That survival sometimes requires becoming something others would call monstrous."

"And what have you become?"

The question hung in the air between them like smoke from a funeral pyre. Mary looked at her hands, remembering all the lives they had taken, all the deaths they had arranged, all the historical forces they had shaped through carefully applied violence.

"I've become what you made me," she said. "Your instrument. Your weapon. The means by which you feed on human fear and suffering."

An Dubhán's laughter was like the sound of winter wind through dead leaves, like the whisper of scavengers picking over ancient battlefields.

"No, Mary," it said gently. "You have become what you chose to become. I offered you power, yes. I showed you opportunities, certainly. But every death you have arranged, every assassination you have performed, every moderate voice you have eliminated, all of it has been your choice, made according to your own understanding of what serves your interests."

The creature moved closer to her, its presence filling the grove with the scent of bog water and ancient decay.

"Do you remember what I told you when we first met? That I was not here to corrupt you but to help you discover what you already were? Forty years later, having shaped the course of European politics through strategic murder, having eliminated dozens of voices that might have prevented the wars and revolutions that are coming, do you finally understand what I meant?"

Mary stared at the ancient thing that had guided her transformation from Irish peasant girl to architect of continental chaos. She had spent decades believing that she was serving An Dubhán's purposes, that her murders were feeding the creature's hunger for fear and death. But now, standing in the place where her violent career had begun, she began to understand something that changed everything.

"I was never your servant," she said slowly. "I was always myself. You didn't corrupt me, you simply showed me what I was capable of becoming when I stopped pretending to be something I wasn't."

An Dubhán smiled with genuine pleasure, like a teacher watching a promising student finally grasp a difficult concept.

"Exactly," it said. "You are Mary Costello, murderess. Not because I made you into that, but because that is what you chose to be when faced with the fundamental questions of existence. Power or submission. Control or victimhood. The strong or the weak."

The creature began to fade, becoming translucent as the autumn light filtered through the oak canopy above them.

"And now," it said as its form dissolved back into the shadows from which it had emerged, "you must decide what comes next. You have spent forty years learning to kill individuals, to eliminate moderate voices, to shape historical events through strategic assassination. But those were merely exercises, Mary. Training for what you were always meant to become."

"Which is?"

"Whatever you choose to be," An Dubhán replied, its voice now barely a whisper in the wind. "You are finally complete, finally fully realized as the thing you were always meant to become. The question is: what will you do with the power you have spent a lifetime accumulating?"

And then the creature was gone, leaving Mary alone in the grove where her story had begun, surrounded by the ghosts of her own past and the weight of possibilities that stretched ahead like an infinite landscape of violence and ambition.

She was home. But home was not the end of her story, it was the place where her real work could finally begin.

Mary Costello stood among the oak trees where she had first killed, where she had first tasted blood, where she had first understood that she was capable of taking whatever she wanted from a world that had tried to deny her agency and power.

Now, finally, she was ready to discover what she truly wanted.

Mary remained in the grove long after An Dubhán's presence had faded, her mind struggling to process the implications of what the creature had revealed. For forty years, she had believed herself to be serving something greater and more terrible than herself. She had taken comfort in the idea that her murders, however numerous and calculated, were performed in service to forces beyond human understanding. It had made her crimes feel purposeful, justified by designs too vast for mortal comprehension.

But now she understood that there had been no grand design, no cosmic purpose, no ancient hunger that required feeding. There had only been Mary Costello, choosing again and again to solve her problems through violence, finding satisfaction in the exercise of power over life and death, discovering that she possessed a talent for killing and deciding to develop that talent to its fullest potential.

She walked to the edge of the grove and looked out across the bog that stretched toward the horizon, its surface reflecting the gray autumn sky like a vast mirror made of still water and accumulated death. How many people had died in this landscape over the centuries? How many bodies had been swallowed by the peat and preserved in its acidic embrace? How many stories of violence and desperation had played out among these hills and valleys before being forgotten by history?

Mary began to laugh, not the bitter sound of someone who had discovered she'd been deceived, but the genuine amusement of someone who had finally understood a joke that had taken decades to appreciate. She had spent her adult life believing that she was a victim of supernatural corruption, a tool wielded by forces beyond her control.

Instead, she had been exactly what she had always appeared to be: a woman who had discovered that she was very good at killing people and had decided to make that skill the foundation of her existence.

"Forty years," she said aloud to the empty landscape. "Forty years of elaborate justifications for doing exactly what I wanted to do anyway."

The realization was liberating in a way that surprised her. She had always carried a small burden of resentment toward An Dubhán, a sense that the creature had stolen something from her when it offered her power in exchange for service. But if the creature had simply been showing her possibilities that were already within her nature to pursue, if every choice had ultimately been her own...

Mary walked back toward the ruins of her childhood cottage, her steps lighter than they had been in decades. She felt like someone who had been carrying a heavy pack for so long that she had forgotten what it felt like to move freely, only to discover that the pack had been empty all along.

The cottage walls still stood, though the roof had long since collapsed and weeds grew through gaps in the stone foundation. Mary pushed through the doorway where no door remained and stood in what had once been the single room where seven people had lived in poverty and desperation and mutual cruelty.

Here was where her father had beaten her, where her brothers had tormented her, where her sister had whispered poison in her ear during the long nights when hunger made sleep impossible. Here was where she had learned that the world was divided into those who inflicted pain and those who suffered it, those who took what they wanted and those who had their desires stripped away by others stronger and more ruthless than themselves.

But here was also where she had made her first choice, not to accept the role of victim that her family had assigned to her, but to become something else, something that would never again be vulnerable to the casual cruelties of those who believed themselves entitled to power over her.

Mary knelt beside the spot where the fireplace had once stood, where her family had gathered for warmth during the cold Irish winters. She began to dig with her hands, clawing through decades of accumulated earth and debris until her fingers found what she was searching for, the smooth stone she had hidden after using it to kill Padraig, the first weapon she had ever wielded, the tool that had transformed her from Mary Costello the victim into Mary Costello the killer.

She lifted the stone from its resting place and held it up to the fading light, noting how unremarkable it appeared, just another piece of Irish granite, worn smooth by water and time, indistinguishable from thousands of others that littered the landscape. But in her hands, it became something more significant: the first instrument of her agency, the means by which she had claimed the right to determine who lived and who died.

"Thank you," she said to the stone, though she was not sure if she was addressing the object itself or the memory of what it had made possible. "Thank you for showing me what I was capable of becoming."

She slipped the stone into her coat pocket, where it settled with a weight that felt familiar and comforting. She had carried more sophisticated weapons in the years since, poisons that could kill without leaving traces, blades forged by master craftsmen, firearms that could end lives from a distance. But this crude piece of granite remained the most important tool she had ever possessed, because it represented the moment when she had stopped being something that happened to and started being something that made things happen.

As evening approached, Mary made her way to the village cemetery where the bodies of her family had been buried decades earlier. The graves were marked with simple wooden crosses that had weathered badly, the names carved into them barely legible after so many seasons of rain and wind. But Mary remembered exactly where each body lay, remembered the weight of earth she had thrown onto crude coffins made from whatever wood the village carpenter could spare.

She stood before her father's grave first, looking down at the mound of earth that contained all that remained of Seamus Costello. He had been a hard man, broken by poverty and loss, who had taken his frustrations out on the child who reminded him most of his failures. But he had also been the man who had taught her, through his violence and neglect, that survival required strength and that strength required the willingness to use whatever weapons were available.

"You made me into what I am," she told his grave. "Not through love or guidance or any of the things fathers are supposed to provide their daughters, but through teaching me that the world is a place where the weak suffer and the strong prosper. You taught me to be strong, even if you never intended to."

She moved to Brigid's grave next, remembering her sister's sharp tongue and cruel disposition, the way she had delighted in reminding Mary that she was unwanted, that she was the reason their mother had died, that she would have been better left to perish with the woman who bore her.

"You taught me that family loyalty is a luxury that only the secure can afford," Mary said to the weathered cross that marked Brigid's resting place. "You showed me that blood relationships are no protection against cruelty, that sisters can be as dangerous as enemies if they see you as a threat to their own survival."

Finally, she came to the section of the cemetery where her brothers lay, Padraig, Cormac, Seamus the younger, Brendan. The men who had seen her not as a sister deserving protection but as prey to be exploited when opportunity arose. They had taught her different lessons: that predators come in familiar forms, that violations of trust are often the most damaging betrayals, that the only reliable protection against those who would harm you is the permanent elimination of the threat they represent.

"Thank you all," Mary said to the gathered graves. "Thank you for showing me exactly what I needed to become to survive in the world you created for me. I learned your lessons well, perhaps too well for your own good."

She spent the night in the ruins of the cottage, wrapped in a cloak she had purchased in the village, listening to the sounds of the Irish countryside and remembering what it had felt like to be the frightened girl who had once lived in this place. But she felt no nostalgia for that earlier version of herself, no regret for the innocence she had lost or the different paths she might have chosen.

Mary Costello had been forged by circumstance, shaped by necessity, and tempered by forty years of violence into exactly what she was meant to be. She was not An Dubhán's creature or the Devil's servant or anyone's tool but her own. She was a killer because she had chosen to be a killer, a shaper of historical forces because she had discovered that she possessed the skill and intelligence to be such a thing.

As dawn broke over the Irish hills, Mary rose from her resting place among the ruins of her childhood and began walking toward the road that would take her back to the larger world. She had work to do, not because some ancient creature commanded it, not because supernatural forces required her service, but because she had spent a lifetime developing capabilities that deserved to be used to their fullest extent.

The wars that were coming to Europe, the revolutions that would reshape nations, the conflicts that would determine the course of human civilization for generations, all of these would happen whether Mary Costello participated in them or not. But with her involvement, they could be guided and shaped and made to serve purposes that satisfied her own understanding of how the world should be arranged.

She was going back to work, but this time she would be working for herself rather than pretending to serve masters who had never existed. She would kill because she was good at killing, manipulate because she enjoyed the exercise of such skills, shape history because she had discovered that she possessed the power to do so.

Mary Costello was finally free, free to be exactly what she had always been beneath all the elaborate justifications and supernatural explanations. She was a murderess, and she was going to enjoy every moment of what came next.

The stone in her pocket weighed nothing at all, but it carried the memory of every choice that had led her to this moment of perfect understanding. She was home, but home was not a place, it was a recognition of her own nature, finally accepted without shame or pretence.

Mary Costello walked away from the bog, away from the graves, away from the ruins of her origins, and back toward the world that awaited her attention. She had never been more herself than she was at this moment, and she had never been more dangerous.

Epilogue

From the private papers of Professor James MacReady, Trinity College Dublin, found among his effects following his death in 1923

I have spent the better part of fifty years studying what the news –"The Bloody Mary Murders"a series of political assassinations that occurred throughout Europe in the middle decades of the nineteenth century. What began as an academic curiosity about patterns in revolutionary violence became something approaching an obsession as I discovered connections that no one else seemed to notice, a thread of deliberate manipulation running through events that historians have always attributed to the natural forces of nationalism and political change.

The woman at the centre of these events used many names: Lady Margaret Sanguinaire in London, Sister Magdalene Caritas in Dublin, Baroness Katarina von Schwarzburg in Vienna, Contessa Elena Ravenna in Rome, Sister Agatha McKenna in Florence. But I have become convinced that all of these identities belonged to a single individual, a woman whose systematic elimination of moderate political voices helped ensure that the unification of both Italy and Germany would be achieved through violence rather than negotiation, whose carefully orchestrated assassinations created the conditions for conflicts that claimed millions of lives.

The evidence for this conclusion is circumstantial but compelling. Physical descriptions that remain consistent despite changes in nationality and social class. Methods of operation that demonstrate increasing sophistication while maintaining certain characteristic elements. Most tellingly, a pattern of targeting that always focused on precisely those individuals whose survival might have prevented or minimised violent conflict.

But it was not until I discovered the manuscript of Father O'Malley, the priest who administered last rites to Mary Costello before her execution in 1849, that I began to understand the true scope of what I was investigating.

According to Father O'Malley's account, Mary Costello confessed to him that she had made a bargain with what she described as "an ancient thing that feeds on death and terror." She claimed to have served this entity for twenty years, arranging murders that appeared random but were actually calculated to maximize fear and despair among the Irish population. Her confession, as recorded by the priest, reads like the ravings of a madwoman—except that every verifiable detail proves to be accurate upon investigation.

Mary Costello was indeed born in a cottage beside Ballymore bog in 1806. Her family did die under the circumstances she described. The murders she confessed to—including several that were never officially connected to her, can be documented through parish records and newspaper accounts. Even her descriptions of the methods she used prove accurate when compared with coroner's reports from the period.

But the most disturbing element of her confession was her claim that death would not end her service to the entity she called An Dubhán. She told Father O'Malley that she expected to be resurrected, to continue her work on a larger scale, to help orchestrate conflicts that would reshape human civilisation according to patterns that served purposes beyond mortal understanding.

I dismissed this as the delusion of a woman driven mad by her own crimes, until I began tracking the activities of those mysterious identities I mentioned earlier, until I realised that someone with Mary Costello's methods and motivations had been active throughout Europe in the decades following her execution.

The woman died on November 15, 1849, her body witnessed by hundreds of spectators and buried in an unmarked grave in Dublin's Glasnevin Cemetery. But six months later, Lady Margaret Sanguinaire appeared in London society with credentials that traced her lineage to families that had never existed and resources that had no identifiable source.

I have devoted my career to rational inquiry, to the careful evaluation of evidence, to explanations that can be tested and verified through scholarly methods. But the deeper I have delved into the mystery of Mary Costello and her apparent continuation under other identities, the more I have been forced to consider possibilities that challenge everything I thought I understood about the nature of life and death.

The political assassinations attributed to various agents throughout the middle nineteenth century follow patterns that suggest coordination by a single intelligence. The elimination of moderate voices in Italy, Germany, and elsewhere created power vacuums that were filled by exactly the kind of extremist elements whose conflicts would prove most destructive to European stability. Someone with intimate knowledge of political psychology and historical forces systematically removed the individuals whose survival might have prevented the wars that defined our modern age.

But even more disturbing than the evidence for supernatural continuation is the possibility that Mary Costello's confessions were accurate in their essential details, that there are forces in this world that feed on human suffering, that use individuals like her as instruments for creating the kinds of conflicts that maximise death and despair.

I write this account knowing that it will never be published during my lifetime, that my colleagues would consider it the product of an ageing mind that has spent too many years contemplating violence and corruption. But I believe that someone must document what I have discovered, must preserve the evidence that connects seemingly unrelated events across decades and continents.

The woman who began as Mary Costello may still be active in the world. The patterns I have identified in historical records suggest that her work continued well beyond the period I have been able to study systematically. If I am correct about her nature and her purposes, then the conflicts that have shaped our modern world, the wars that have claimed millions of lives, the revolutions that have overturned the established order, the ethnic hatreds that poison entire regions, may not be the natural consequences of human ambition and political development.

They may be the carefully orchestrated results of strategic murders performed by someone who learned to see individual deaths as brush strokes in a much larger painting, someone who discovered that history itself could be shaped by those willing to pay the price in blood that such shaping requires.

I have spent my life studying the forces that drive human conflict, trying to understand how rational beings can repeatedly choose destruction over cooperation, violence over negotiation, war over peace. Mary Costello's story suggests an answer that is more terrifying than any I had previously considered: perhaps we do not choose these things at all. Perhaps they are chosen for us by intelligences that understand our weaknesses better than we understand them ourselves.

If this manuscript is ever discovered and read, I hope that whoever finds it will have the wisdom to recognise both its importance and its danger. The evidence I have collected should be preserved, but it should also be approached with the understanding that some knowledge carries risks that extend far beyond academic reputation.

Mary Costello claimed to serve something that had been old when the world was young, something that would continue its work long after every human soul had been consumed by the darkness it represented. If she was telling the truth, if such entities truly exist and truly use human agents to orchestrate the conflicts that feed their hunger, then understanding them may be our only hope of breaking free from patterns that have trapped our species in cycles of violence for millennia.

But understanding them may also mean attracting their attention, becoming targets ourselves for the kind of elimination that removes inconvenient voices from the world's stage.

I am an old man now, my health failing, my time limited. I have spent decades gathering evidence that points toward conclusions most people would consider impossible. I do not expect to live long enough to see whether that evidence proves useful to anyone else. But I have done what I could to preserve it, to create a record that might help others recognise the true nature of the forces that shape our world.

The woman who called herself Mary Costello understood something that the rest of us prefer to ignore: that individual choices, however small, can have consequences that ripple across centuries. She chose to become a killer when she was fourteen years old, standing in a grove of oak trees beside an Irish bog. That choice, and all the choices that followed from it, may have determined the course of human history in ways that we are only beginning to comprehend.

I pray that I am wrong about her continued existence, wrong about the supernatural forces I believe guided her work, wrong about the possibility that such entities continue to manipulate human affairs through agents we cannot identify or stop.

But if I am right, then God help us all. Because Mary Costello was not the disease, she was merely the symptom of something far older and more implacable than any evil the human imagination has conceived.

The real horror is not that such people exist, but that they may be exactly what they appear to be: the inevitable product of forces that have been shaping human development since our species first learned to make war upon itself.

Professor James MacReady

Trinity College Dublin

December 1922

Found among Professor MacReady's papers was a single additional note, written in a different hand on expensive stationery:

"Dear Professor MacReady - Your research was admirably thorough, though not quite complete. You were correct about more things than you realised, and incorrect about several details that might have provided you with comfort had you understood them properly. Do not concern yourself overmuch with the implications of what you discovered. History has its own momentum now, and individuals, however gifted, are merely components in machinery too vast for any single mind to comprehend. Your death will appear entirely natural, as will the disappearance of your research materials. But your work will not be entirely wasted. Someone must keep records, after all. With sincere appreciation for your dedication to the truth. - M.C."

Professor MacReady died peacefully in his sleep three days later. His research materials were never found.